ESSENTIALS OF
NEUROPSYCHOLOGICAL REHABILITATION

Also Available

The Brain Injury Rehabilitation Workbook
Edited by Rachel Winson, Barbara A. Wilson,
and Andrew Bateman

Memory Rehabilitation: Integrating Theory and Practice
Barbara A. Wilson

ESSENTIALS OF NEUROPSYCHOLOGICAL REHABILITATION

BARBARA A. WILSON

SHAI BETTERIDGE

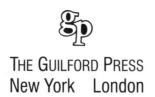

THE GUILFORD PRESS
New York   London

LIMITED DUPLICATION LICENSE

These materials are intended for use only by qualified mental health professionals.

The publisher grants to individual purchasers of this book nonassignable permission
to reproduce all materials for which photocopying permission is specifically granted in
a footnote. This license is limited to you, the individual purchaser, for personal use or
use with individual patients. This license does not grant the right to reproduce these
materials for resale, redistribution, electronic display, or any other purposes (including
but not limited to books, pamphlets, articles, video- or audiotapes, blogs, file-sharing sites,
Internet or intranet sites, and handouts or slides for lectures, workshops, webinars, or
therapy groups, whether or not a fee is charged). Permission to reproduce these materials
for these and any other purposes must be obtained in writing from the Permissions
Department of Guilford Publications.

The authors have checked with sources believed to be reliable in their efforts to provide
information that is complete and generally in accord with the standards of practice that are
accepted at the time of publication. However, in view of the possibility of human error or
changes in behavioral, mental health, or medical sciences, neither the authors, nor the editor
and publisher, nor any other party who has been involved in the preparation or publication
of this work warrants that the information contained herein is in every respect accurate or
complete, and they are not responsible for any errors or omissions or the results obtained from
the use of such information. Readers are encouraged to confirm the information contained in
this book with other sources.

Library of Congress Cataloging-in-Publication Data is available from
the publisher.

ISBN 978-1-4625-4073-0 (paper)
ISBN 978-1-4625-4074-7 (hardcover)

About the Authors

Barbara A. Wilson, OBE, PhD, a clinical neuropsychologist, is founder of the Oliver Zangwill Centre for Neuropsychological Rehabilitation in Ely, Cambridgeshire, United Kingdom. She has worked in brain injury rehabilitation since the 1970s. Dr. Wilson has published 26 books, over 300 journal articles and book chapters, and eight neuropsychological tests, and is editor of the journal *Neuropsychological Rehabilitation*. She has won many awards for her work, including five lifetime achievement awards, the Ramón y Cajal Award from the International Neuropsychiatric Association, and the M. B. Shapiro Award from the British Neuropsychological Society. She is past president of the British Neuropsychological Society and the International Neuropsychological Society, and is currently president of the Encephalitis Society and on the management committee of the World Federation for NeuroRehabilitation. Dr. Wilson is a Fellow of the British Psychological Society, the Academy of Medical Sciences, and the Academy of Social Sciences. She is an honorary professor at the University of Hong Kong, the University of Sydney, and the University of East Anglia, United Kingdom, and holds honorary degrees from the University of East Anglia and the University of Córdoba in Argentina.

Shai Betteridge, PsychD, CPsychol, PGDip (Clinical Neuropsychology), is Head of the Clinical Neuropsychology and Clinical Health Psychology Department at St. George's Hospital in London, and Clinical Lead for The Wolfson Neurorehabilitation Centre's Cognitive Rehabilitation Program. She is a chartered clinical psychologist with the British Psychological Society, a member of its Division of Neuropsychology's Specialist Register of Clinical Neuropsychologists, and a registered practitioner psychologist with the U.K. Health and Care Professions Council. Dr. Betteridge has worked in various areas related to research on and the application of neuropsychology and neuropsychological rehabilitation. She also has a keen interest in national government agendas that have an impact on the field of neuropsychological rehabilitation and participates in several working parties committed to quality improvement and excellence. Dr. Betteridge is a Care Quality Commission specialist inspector for neuropsychology services, is proactively involved in providing core teaching modules in neuropsychology for the Clinical Psychology training courses in London, and is a supervisor and oral examiner for the U.K. Qualification in Clinical Neuropsychology.

Preface

This book explains our views on the essential principles of neuropsychological rehabilitation (NR), which, above all, is concerned with improving the lives of people with brain injury and their families.

A distinguishing feature of a profession is that the work of its members is informed by theory, current research, and innovation in the workplace. Essential information engendered during this process is usually passed on to members of the profession by specialized literature in the form of books, research papers, and journals. The authors of this book regard it as rooted in this process as we attempt to pass on to readers the essential "nuts and bolts" of NR as it stands currently and *at its cutting edge throughout the world*. We are, above all, practitioners who also happen to be researchers, writers, and teachers, who have lectured at both a national and international level. We are aware that, while the essentials we discuss in this book may be broadly relevant to our audience, they also have to be tempered by the professional circumstances in which different members of that audience are working. At times, these circumstances themselves will be influenced greatly by national and even local sets of conditions and different restrictions (including financial) that affect the way professionals *can* work. Whether you are, say, working in an experienced and technically brilliant clinic in the United States, or practicing in a hut in Botswana, we hope that what we have to say is relevant to discussions you have with colleagues, informs debate, and even at times stimulates argument. It is also important for us to stress that NR can be cost effective over the long term, and we cite research that shows this to be true, quoting substantial evidence that there are ways of creating cheaper methods of rehabilitation in society, as well as in hospitals. Our arguments run counter to those that would emphasize the difficulties of costs involved in rehabilitation and time strictures, and to those who might use these so-called difficulties as a way of justifying lack of progress. Another feature of a profession is that it remains positive in the face of social, financial, and political difficulties: We should always be aiming for a brighter side that leads to progress.

We discuss varying definitions of NR, providing a historical account as well as contemporary debate, explaining the difference between recovery and rehabilitation, and arguing that all rehabilitation should eventually provide optimum levels of well-being. We concede that NR requires a broad theoretical basis and examine the many theories that influence the design of NR programs. We concur that good theories should teach us to approach our treatment and assessment with as many questions as answers. We evaluate both standardized and behavioral assessments, making the case for both to be included in the neuropsychologist's toolbox.

We expect our audience to include neuropsychologists, clinical psychologists, occupational therapists, physiotherapists, social workers, nurses, medical doctors, speech and language therapists, patients, and families, and the rehabilitation programs we describe are the result of consultation among patients, their families, and professional staff, all of whom need to be members of the same rehabilitation team. We accept that rehabilitation goals should be realistic and deal with real-life issues, rather than artificial goals more attuned to the laboratory. We argue strongly that NR programs should be holistic, dealing with emotional, behavioral, and cognitive issues, some of which might be assisted by modern technology whenever appropriate. Indeed, modern technology features strongly in our consideration of future developments.

At times, we refer to the work that goes on at the Oliver Zangwill Centre in the United Kingdom, founded by Barbara A. Wilson and involved in NR and research, many examples of which are cited in this book. We also use examples from the Wolfson Neurorehabilitation Centre, St. George's Hospital, in London, where Shai Betteridge works, as well as examples of good practice from the United States. We evaluate holistic programs, group therapy, and individual therapy. Goals at the Oliver Zangwill Centre include increased awareness, the promotion of understanding, cognitive rehabilitation, the development of compensatory skills, and vocational counseling. We consider the provision of a therapeutic milieu, meaningful functional activity, shared understanding, the application of psychological therapies, the consideration of emotional issues, the use of compensatory strategies, and working with families.

Acknowledgments

We wish to thank Jill Winegardner, Jessica Fish, and Sanjay Sunak for permission to use the formulation diagrams in Chapter 5; Gary Hayward for permission to use the case study about him; Jose David Jaramillo for permission to use his case study; the Redgrave family for permission to use the case study on the late Corin Redgrave; Jessica Fish for help with the references and for her moral support; Rochelle Serwator of The Guilford Press for persuading us to write the book and for her support throughout; and Mick Wilson for proofreading and helpful comments throughout the writing process.

Contents

CHAPTER 1

What Is Neuropsychological Rehabilitation?

Introduction

Neuropsychology is the study of the relationship between brain and behavior; it is concerned with how the brain affects behavior, emotion, and cognition. Rehabilitation is a process whereby people are enabled to return to as normal a life as possible following illness or disease. Neuropsychological rehabilitation (NR) is a process whereby people disabled by injury or disease work together with professional staff, relatives, and members of the wider community to achieve their optimum physical, psychological, social, and vocational well-being. NR is offered not only to patients who are expected to recover, partially or completely, but to all patients with long-term problems (Donaghy, 2011). There are increasing numbers of people requiring NR due to medical advances in recent decades (Noggle, Dean, & Barisa, 2013). NR is not synonymous with recovery (if by recovery we mean getting back to what one was like before the injury or illness); nor is it the same as treatment, which is something we *do* to people or *give* to people when, for instance, we prescribe drugs or administer surgery. Instead, it is a two-way interactive process concerned with the amelioration of cognitive, emotional, psychosocial, and behavioral deficits caused by an insult to the brain. Donaghy (2011) reminds us that the focus of NR is on the patient as a person, and how his or her goals relate to social functioning, as well as health and well-being. As Ylvisaker and Feeney (2000) argue, rehabilitation involves personally meaningful themes, activities, settings, and interactions. Given such due status, we should not set goals that lack meaning for the patient, such as "improve performance on a memory test." Nor should we set goals that are vague, such as "improve memory functioning"; or goals that are highly unlikely to be achievable, such as "restore memory functioning."

As well as making life better for patients with brain injuries and their families, NR also makes economic sense. There is plenty of evidence to show that neuropsychological rehabilitation is clinically effective. Cicerone and his colleagues, for example, in a meta-analysis, found that NR programs can improve community integration, functional independence, and productivity, even for patients who are many years postinjury (Cicerone et al., 2011). Van Heugten, Gregorio, and Wade (2012) investigated 95 randomized controlled trials carried out between 1980 and 2010 and concluded that there is a large body of evidence to support the efficacy of cognitive rehabilitation. Although rehabilitation may be expensive in the short term, there is evidence that it is cost-effective in the long term (Wilson, Winegardner, & Ashworth, 2014). The costs of *not* rehabilitating people with brain injury are considerable given the fact that many are young, with a relatively normal life expectancy (McMillan & Greenwood, 1993). Substantial economic benefits, as well as familial and social improvements, make it almost impossible to deny the advantages to be gained by "comprehensive-holistic neuropsychologic rehabilitation, recommended to improve post-acute participation and quality of life after moderate or severe TBI [traumatic brain injury]" (Cicerone et al., 2011). A further issue is raised by Noggle et al. (2013) when they argue that cognitive deficits, as a major part of NR, are particularly troubling, as they can affect adaptability and are not recognized by the public. These authors also claim that the traditional medical rehabilitation model is inappropriate for dealing with many of the deficits, and that neuropsychology is better placed to do this. This makes sense, as NR is not a one-time treatment but requires a committed, comprehensive, and coherent alliance among patient, family, health service staff, and possibly other interested parties such as employers, teachers, and social workers. Fundamental issues arising from the above definitions will form the basis of what is to follow in this book.

A Brief History
of Neuropsychological Rehabilitation

According to Brewer-Mixon and Callum (2013), NR can be traced back to ancient man and his attempts to cure ills through trepanning, in which a hole was bored into the skull to let out evil spirits. Wilson (2017) explains that one of the earliest known descriptions of the treatment of brain injury is from an Egyptian papyrus of 2,500–3,000 years ago. This was discovered by Edwin Smith in Luxor in 1862 (recounted by Walsh, 1987). It describes the treatment of 27 brain trauma cases. The document contains the first known descriptions of the cranial structures, the meninges, the external surface of the brain, the cerebrospinal fluid, and the intracranial pulsations. The word "brain" appears here for the first time in any language. The ancient Egyptians appeared to have a level of knowledge surpassing that of Hippocrates, who lived 1,000 years later. As Brewer-Mixon and Callum (2013) remind us, however, people in the later Greek civilization were misled because of the popular cultural or religious beliefs of Aristotle's time, when, for example, Aristotle himself believed that the heart was the seat of mental functions. We learn, too, from Brewer-Mixon and Callum, of the much later anatomical contributions of Vesalius and Willis, and that Wernicke was among the first to recognize that brain functions resulted from a series of regions interconnected by neural pathways.

A few reports describing treatment appeared over the centuries, including a case of Paul Broca's (1865, reported in Boake, 1996). Broca was treating an adult patient who was no longer able to read words aloud. This patient was first taught to read letters, then syllables, before combining syllables into words. He failed, however, to learn to read words of more than one syllable so the treatment was then switched to a whole-word approach and he learned to recognize a number of them.

Modern rehabilitation, as we understand it today, however, began in World War I because more soldiers with gunshot injuries, including those with penetrating head wounds, survived as a result of improvements in medicine and surgery. This led to the setting up of dedicated brain injury rehabilitation centers for the first time (Boake, 1996). The most important and influential person from that era was Kurt Goldstein, a German neurologist and psychiatrist who was a pioneer in modern neuropsychology. He treated soldiers at the front before sending them to a milieu therapeutic department in Frankfurt, where evaluations were performed by psychologists. The Frankfurt center included a residential hospital, a psychological evaluation unit, and a special workshop for patients to practice and be evaluated in vocational skills (Poser, Kohler, & Schönle, 1996).

Goldstein made specific recommendations about therapy for impairments of speech, reading, and writing (Goldstein, 1919, 1942; Boake, 1996). He can be regarded as the forerunner of holistic rehabilitation when he argued that we should look at the whole aspect of a situation and not one isolated part such as, for example, word-finding difficulties. Ben-Yishay and Diller (2010) say that the importance of Goldstein to the practice of holistic rehabilitation cannot be overemphasized. Poppelreuter (1917/1990) was another German working in World War I, who wrote the first book on brain injury rehabilitation. Both these men were in favor of a functional approach, with Poppelreuter arguing that the first and main goal of therapy was the restoration of skills to enable people to best cope in everyday life. Sadly, wars tend to lead to developments in rehabilitation, so another move forward came in World War II when Luria was probably the most important contributor to developments in NR, although Zangwill from the United Kingdom and Cranich, Wepman, and Aita from the United States were also influential (see Wilson, 2017, for a summary). Luria (1979) believed that psychological research should be for the benefit of humankind and argued that we should look at the patient within the context of his or her social context.

Yet another armed conflict that had a big influence on brain injury rehabilitation was the Yom Kippur War of 1973. Yehuda Ben-Yishay, an American Israeli, was invited back to Israel after the war to work on a joint project of the Israeli Ministry of Defense and the New York University Institute of Rehabilitation Medicine. A day treatment course, influenced by the work of Goldstein, was established in 1975 in Tel Aviv, and can be considered the forerunner of holistic programs. Ben-Yishay (1996) describes how it was initiated, explaining that he had already treated some Israeli soldiers sent to New York for rehabilitation prior to the Yom Kippur War and realized that a different kind of approach to the rehabilitation then provided was needed. About 250 soldiers sustained a brain injury in the Yom Kippur War and had received good physical care but were "unable to resume productive lives, primarily because of residual neurobehavioral, cognitive and psychological problems" (pp. 327–328). With backing from people in New York and Israel, the therapeutic community and holistic treatment style was born. The holistic approach is described more fully in Chapter 9.

In more recent times, people who have been influential in NR include Diller in New York, who devised the first program to be called "cognitive rehabilitation" (Diller, 1976); Prigatano (1986), influenced by Ben-Yishay, who opened a center in Oklahoma and then moved to Phoenix, Arizona; Christensen, who designed a holistic program in Copenhagen, Denmark (Christensen & Teasdale, 1995); and Wilson and her colleagues, who opened the Oliver Zangwill Centre in Cambridgeshire, England, in 1996 (Wilson et al., 2000).

Recovery from Acquired Brain Injury

Recovery usually applies to a return to a normal state of health but most people with severe brain injury will not completely regain all the functions, abilities, and skills they had prior to a brain injury. Jennet and Bond (1975) interpreted recovery as the resumption of normal life even though there may be minor neurological or psychological deficits; and such a state is possible for some survivors of TBI.

"Recovery" has also been defined as the diminution of impairments in behavioral or physiological functions over time (Marshall, 1985), which is likely to occur for the majority of patients. Perhaps the best way to interpret recovery for survivors of brain injury is provided by Kolb (1995), himself a survivor of a stroke, who indicated that recovery typically involves *partial* recovery of function together with *substitution* of function. This is probably the definition of recovery that most closely reflects the situation for the majority of people with brain damage.

Natural Recovery

Fasotti (2017) argues that the brain is capable of self-repair after an injury depending on a number of causes. Brain damage resulting from TBI can be due to both primary and secondary causes. "Primary damage" is that which occurs as a direct result of the accident or insult such as contusions or shearing of axons. "Secondary damage" is due to complications arising from the initial injury such as reduced blood pressure or infections. If secondary damage is avoided through expert medical care, then the final outcome or recovery is maximized. In the words of Miller, Pentland, and Berrol (1990), "the final outcome of any patient who suffers head injury is governed by three groups of factors: the pre-injury status of the brain, the total amount of damage done to the brain by the impact of the head injury (primary damage), and the cumulative effect of the secondary pathological damage to the already injured brain" (p. 21). Secondary damage may result in more permanent disability than primary damage even though it is, at least potentially, avoidable (Daisley, Tams, & Kischka, 2009).

Although recovery from TBI is variable, far from uniform, and may, in some individuals, continue for years (Millis et al., 2001), most survivors undergo some, and often considerable, recovery. This is likely to be fairly rapid in the early weeks and months postinjury, followed by a slower recovery that can continue for many years. A similar pattern may be seen following other kinds of nonprogressive injury including stroke, encephalitis, and hypoxia. In these latter cases, however, the recovery process may last months rather than years (Wilson, 2003a).

Factors Influencing Recovery

A number of factors influence the extent of recovery, some of which we can do nothing about once the damage has occurred. These include the age of the person at the time of insult, the severity of damage, the location of damage, the status of undamaged areas of the brain, and the premorbid cognitive status of the brain. Other factors such as motivation, family support systems, and the quality of rehabilitation available can be manipulated. We now consider three major factors that may influence recovery, namely, age, gender, and cognitive reserve.

In 1940, Kennard showed that young primates with lesions in the motor and premotor cortex exhibited sparing and partial recovery of motor function. Her findings came to be known as the "Kennard principle" and they probably encouraged the fairly widespread belief that children recover better than adults from an insult to the brain (Johnson, Rose, Brooks, & Eyers, 2003). Even Kennard, however, recognized that such sparing did not always occur and that some problems became worse over time. Several later studies have shown that younger children fare worse than older children (Forsyth et al., 2001; Hessen, Nestvold, & Anderson, 2007), and suggest that younger children, particularly those below the age of 2 years, fare worse in the long term than older children. Those studies suggesting the opposite (Montour-Proulx et al., 2004) or suggest no difference (Mosch, Max, & Tranel, 2005) may be looking at children with focal rather than diffuse lesions.

Age, then, is just one factor in the recovery process that has to be considered alongside other perhaps more important factors such as whether the lesion is focal or diffuse (Levin, 2003), the severity of the insult, and the time since acquisition of the function under consideration. Thus, someone who has just learned to read at the time of the insult is more likely to show reading deficits than someone who learned to read many years before.

What about gender? In 1987, Attella, Nattinville, and Stein (1987) suggested that female animals may be protected against the effects of brain injury at certain stages of their cycle due to the effects of estrogen and progesterone. This was confirmed by Roof and Hall (2000). Potentially important for rehabilitation (Stein, 2007), progesterone has been given to survivors of TBI with some suggestion that this leads to a better outcome (Ratcliff et al., 2007). In addition, some studies have looked at the long-term outcomes for females and males following TBI. The findings are contradictory with, for example, Ratcliff et al. (2007) suggesting that females do better than males, while other studies suggest the opposite (Farace & Alves, 2000; Ponsford et al., 2008). The Ponsford et al. study controlled for Glasgow Coma Scale score, age, and cause of injury; they found that females had both a lower rate of survival and a lower rate of good outcome at 6 months postinjury. The authors thought this might be due to the fact that more females died in the early stages. In general, they found no evidence that women did better and some evidence that they did worse than males.

People whose brain injuries are in similar locations, of the same severity, and of the same extent may, nevertheless, have very different problems and outcomes. This led to the concept of "cognitive reserve," which is the third factor to be considered in the understanding of recovery from brain injury. The principle of cognitive reserve suggests that people with more education and higher intelligence may show less impairment than those with poor education and low intelligence. Stern (2007) suggests that individuals with high intelligence may process tasks in a more efficient way. Consequently, in cases of Alzheimer's disease, task impairment manifests itself later in the disease in people with such cognitive reserve. Stern also reminds us that most clinicians are aware of the fact that any insult of the same severity can produce profound damage in one patient and minimal damage in another. This may also explain differences in recovery following non-progressive brain injury because, as Symonds said in an often-quoted remark, "It is not only the kind of head injury that matters but the kind of head" (1937, p. 1092).

According to Stern (2007), although there is no direct relationship between the degree of damage and the clinical manifestation of that damage, there are two separate models of cognitive reserve. One is a passive model, which depends on the number of neurons possessed by an individual, or the person's brain size; while the other is an active model in which the brain activates its cognitive-processing strategies or compensatory techniques in order to deal with damage.

Bigler (2007) believes that the passive model of cognitive reserve helps to explain not only the initial recovery from TBI but also recovery across the lifespan. This passive model allows us to understand why there is an increased risk of dementia in survivors of TBI. With regard to the active model of cognitive reserve, Schutz (2007) offers support in the description of nine highly successful survivors of severe TBI. These were far more successful than their peers in cognitive, academic, and social achievements because they implemented procedures to minimize the impact of their deficits.

How Does Recovery Occur?

We still have much to learn about the process of recovery. It probably involves different biological processes including plasticity of the central nervous system (CNS), such as the reorganization of the preexisting network and axonal sprouting (Taupin, 2006). Changes seen in the first few minutes, for example, after a mild head injury with no permanent structural damage, are probably due to the resolution of temporary dysfunction such as when the structures are stunned but not destroyed. This is akin to what Robertson and Murre (1999) refer to when they say that plastic reorganization may occur because of a rapidly occurring alteration in synaptic activity taking place over seconds or minutes. Recovery after several days is more likely to be due to resolution of temporary structural abnormalities such as edema or vascular disruption (Jennett, 1990), or to the depression of metabolic enzyme activity (Whyte, 1990). Recovery after months or years is even less well understood. Regeneration, diaschisis, and plasticity are three possible ways this can occur (Stein & Hoffman, 2003). Fasotti (2017), however, suggests that although diaschisis is one mechanism, functional network recovery and behavioral adaptation may also explain recovery from brain injury.

"Regeneration" refers to the regrowth of neurons following brain damage. For regeneration to take place, it is necessary for new cells and axons to survive and integrate into existing neural networks (Johansson, 2007). Logan, Oliver, and Berry (2007) believe that neurons do begin to regrow initially but this ceases as scarring of fibers occurs, preventing reconnection of severed neuronal pathways. Consequently, functional recovery from such injuries is poor. Voss et al. (2006), however, argue that axonal regrowth may take place many years after severe brain injury. They report one patient who regained functional speech despite being in a minimally conscious state for 19 years.

Cell implantation could also lead to regeneration; several studies have addressed this possibility. Ma, Zhang, and Li (2007) found that bone marrow stromal cells can promote recovery from TBI when injected directly into the brain or the cerebrospinal fluid or the bloodstream. The authors caution that there are many problems to be solved, as recognized by Parr, Tator, and Keating (2007) who say that the transplantation of bone marrow cells is unlikely to be a major factor in recovery from TBI. They believe that other factors such as neuroprotection and enriched environments play a greater role. Taupin (2006) claims that after TBI and stroke new neuronal cells are generated at the sites of injury where they replace some of the degenerated nerve cells indicating that the CNS is attempting to regenerate itself. The widely held belief for many years was that cerebral plasticity is severely restricted in the adult human brain. This is no longer tenable, as there is now sufficient evidence to show that some regeneration of brain cells does occur after brain damage. Taupin (2006) says that there is a great deal of neurological recovery in the months and years following brain damage despite frequently occurring permanent structural damage. What is less clear, however, is the extent to which regeneration can lead to useful gains in coping with real-life problems.

"Diaschisis" is a term first used by von Monakow (1915). It assumes that damage to a specific area of the brain can result in neural shock or disruption elsewhere in the brain. This could be adjacent to the site of the primary insult or much further away (Miller, 1984). In either case, the shock follows a particular neural route. Robertson and Murre (1999, p. 547) interpret diaschisis as "a weakening of synaptic connections between the damaged and undamaged sites." Because cells in the two areas are no longer firing together, synaptic connectivity between them is weakened, resulting in the lowering of functioning in the undamaged but partly disconnected remote site.

Plasticity is the third mechanism by which recovery can take place. Although in the neuroscience literature the term "plasticity" refers to both positive and negative responses to environmental factors and to insults to the brain, in brain injury rehabilitation the term refers to anatomical reorganization whereby an undamaged part of the brain can take over the functioning of a damaged area. In Duffau's (2006) words, cerebral plasticity is "the dynamic potential of the brain to reorganize itself during ontogeny, learning, or following damage" (p. 885). Until recently, this idea was discredited as an explanation for recovery in adults, although views are now changing. Bütefisch (2004) suggests that the human adult brain retains the ability to reorganize itself throughout life. Cecatto and Chadi (2007) suggest that behavioral experience and neuronal stimulation play a part in modifying the functional organization of remaining cortical tissue and can lead to clinical improvements.

"Functional network recovery" refers to the spontaneous cognitive and behavioral recovery achieved by a reorganization of intact neural circuits (Fasotti, 2017). This is based on the suggestion of Luria (1963), who questioned whether a remodeling of neuronal networks could underlie functional recovery. This has been confirmed in the last few years by functional imaging studies, which have shown that cerebral reorganization can result in shifts of activity within the brain (Fasotti, 2017). Cerebral reorganization, however, has mostly been shown to occur in studies of language and motor deficits (Fasotti, 2017).

Behavioral adaptation mechanism has also been considered as an explanation for recovery. This refers to the occurrence of spontaneous behavioral compensations without specific training and entails the unintentional use of different systems when carrying out a task. An example would be patients with recovered neglect bisecting a line accurately but making a much wider arc with their arm to do this compared to control subjects (Goodale, Milner, Jakobson, & Carey, 1990).

Robertson (2002) suggests that recovery is rapid for deficits that are subserved by multiple circuits such as unilateral neglect and slowest for deficits that are subserved by a more limited number of circuits such as hemianopia because fewer alternative pathways are available to take over the functioning of the damaged pathways. This could be the reason why language functions appear to show better recovery over time than memory functions (Kolb, 1995).

Robertson and Murre (1999) believe that two mechanisms can cause plastic reorganization. The first is due to a rapidly occurring alteration in synaptic activity taking place over seconds or minutes, while the second is because of structural changes taking place over days and weeks. The authors posit that some people show spontaneous recovery with no specific intervention; others show very little recovery, even over a period of years and compensatory approaches should be used with these people; still others show reasonably good recovery provided they receive rehabilitation. This is described as the "assisted recovery group" and can address issues of plasticity. It is also believed by Robertson and Murre that the severity of the brain damage determines which group people belong to. Thus, mild lesions result in spontaneous recovery; people with moderate lesions benefit from assisted recovery, and those with severe lesions require the compensatory approach.

Although there may be some truth in this, the idea may be too simplistic because the location of the lesion almost certainly plays a role in rehabilitation. For example, people with mild lesions in the frontal lobes could be more disadvantaged in terms of recovery than people with severe lesions in the left anterior temporal lobe. The former group might have attention, planning, and organization problems precluding them from gaining the maximum benefit from the rehabilitation offered, whereas the latter group, with language problems, could show considerable plasticity by transferring some of the language functions to the right hemisphere (Wilson, 2003a). All those who do not show spontaneous recovery, however, require rehabilitation. This may focus on attempts to restore lost functioning or to help people compensate for their everyday problems or, as is often the case in rehabilitation, a mixture of the two.

More recently, hyperbaric oxygen therapy (HBOT) has been advocated to aid recovery from acquired brain injury (ABI; Huang & Obenaus, 2011). Used most often for people with multiple sclerosis (Bennett & Heard, 2010), this is a form of treatment in which oxygen is administered under increased pressure in a specially designed chamber, thus increasing the amount of oxygen in the blood, brain, and bodily tissues. It is believed that, together with other therapies, HBOT acts as a protective agent for TBI patients and one that may improve long-term outcomes (Huang & Obenaus, 2011). It has also been used for people following a stroke (Ding, Tong, Lu, & Peng, 2014) and carbon monoxide poisoning (Buckley et al., 2011). There are, however, conflicting reports of its efficacy, with some, including Bennett and Heard (2010), arguing that certain individuals may benefit but it is not recommended as a routine treatment. Others claim improvement for people with TBI (Sahni et al., 2012). These authors suggest that HBOT may revive idling neurons. Buckley et al. (2011) recommend it for people who survive carbon monoxide poisoning. A Cochrane Review, however, published in 2012 (Bennett, Trytko, & Jonker) is more skeptical, claiming that while HBOT, used in conjunction with other therapies, may reduce the risk of death and improve the final GCS in people with a TBI, there is little evidence that the survivors have a good outcome. In contrast, a randomized controlled trial (Boussi-Gross et al., 2013) suggests that HBOT can improve functioning in people with a mild TBI several years after the injury. Hu et al. (2016) list the options for future research. A recent review of 12 randomized controlled studies (Crawford et al., 2017) says that although some studies are methodologically flawed, there is some evidence indicating that for those who have sustained a mild TBI, HBOT may be beneficial as a reasonably safe additional therapy. In the face of these findings, we await further details of HBOT as a therapy for survivors of brain injury.

When Does Recovery Occur?

While the empirical evidence is largely clear about the value of neurorehabilitation after ABI, there is considerable debate about how long neurorehabilitation should last for and how to assess "rehabilitation potential" (Burton et al., 2015; Turner-Stokes et al., 2015). Most of the high-impact research in this area is conducted during the acute and early postacute recovery period, when participants can be more easily identified following their hospital admission. The pursuit of Category A/Level 1 evidence in research has meant that tangible outcome measures are favored over the softer psychological factors, because the latter are harder to control and compare. Consequently, the evidence base is artificially biased toward supporting the role of physical rehabilitation early in recovery (cf. Turner-Stokes et al., 2006). There is generally a lack of good-quality longitudinal evidence about recovery from ABI, but it is noteworthy that in a retrospective analysis of service use up to 17 years post-TBI, psychosocial disability was a better predictor of neurorehabilitation service use than physical or cognitive disability alone (Hodgkinson et al., 2000).

The medical profession has long been a proponent of the view that it can predict prognosis following illness; consequently, following ABI, patients frequently expect health professionals to be able to answer the question, "When will I get better?" In our clinical experience, during the acute and postacute phases of recovery it is very difficult to predict with any certainty, when, or how much, someone will recover. While it is widely acknowledged that survivors of TBI generally have better but more varied recovery trajectories than survivors of hypoxic brain injury, who tend to plateau quickly and have poorer outcomes (Cullen & Weisz, 2011), mediating factors such as the patient's cognitive reserve and the family's motivation and determination to facilitate change can have an impact on recovery (e.g., see Case Study 1.1 below).

Clinicians generally accept the conclusion that their ability to distinguish between those with a poor prognosis versus those with a slower recovery trajectory is inadequate, and therefore objective measures such as goal attainment are favored to guide decision making (Turner-Stokes, Williams, & Johnson, 2009). As a result, patients who are not making demonstrable changes in rehabilitation are deemed to have "no rehabilitation potential" and are generally transferred to long-term residential and/or nursing home placements. Fundamentally, such decisions are taken to ensure access to the limited resource of neurorehabilitation inpatient beds is allocated to those most able to make use of them.

In our experience, patients can continue to recover from ABI many years after the event (see Case Study 1.2 below), and often some years after health services have concluded that there is little or no "rehabilitation potential" (McMillan & Herbert, 2004; Wilson, Dhamapurkar, & Rose, 2016). In cases where recovery of function has occurred after a protracted period of slow or static recovery, factors such as the individual's mood, motivation, personal determination, self-efficacy, and level of social and emotional support appear to play a large role in facilitating change in addition to physiological spontaneous recovery (Wilson et al., 2016). There is usually also some element of slow-stream rehabilitation available to the patient. As the "soft" factors detailed here cannot be identified in the early stages of rehabilitation, it becomes difficult to predict who would benefit from slow-stream rehabilitation, and therefore it seems only those with families or treating teams who can advocate for them currently receive such placements.

Arguably, slow-stream rehabilitation should be available for those with the most severe disabilities over the long term, as it is essential to good disability management; and if late spontaneous recovery is going to occur, access to rehabilitation will ensure this opportunity is harnessed. However, due to the way health services are funded in Western societies (i.e., via health insurance companies or cash-strapped

National Health Services [NHS]), rehabilitation is primarily offered in the first few years after the index event. This has led to a fallacy about the recovery trajectory after ABI, which patients often quote, that is, "The majority of recovery occurs in the first 2 years after ABI." Health services often fund rehabilitation in accordance with this time scale because of resource issues, but there is no hard evidence to support this arbitrary cut-off point (Millis et al., 2001). Unfortunately, well-meaning medical staff often state this trajectory to patients early on in their rehabilitation journey to help them understand that recovery is a long-term process; but it becomes a point of significant distress to patients, especially when they reach this milestone and they have not achieved the rate of recovery they desire. This can trigger a mental health breakdown, which in turn reduces rehabilitation engagement and potential for change.

It is also the case that patients often lack insight into their deficits and therefore disengage from rehabilitation at the time when they are being offered it because they have not yet been exposed to such deficits in everyday life. After multiple failed attempts at community reintegration they come to the realization that there is a problem and may only be ready to engage in rehabilitation several years after the index event. Sadly, it is difficult to obtain funding for rehabilitation at these times and so it becomes a self-fulfilling prophecy (i.e., the majority of rehabilitation occurs in the first 2 years), as patients find it difficult to access NR beyond this 2-year point.

In reality, changes in functioning can continue to occur for many years postinjury, both positive and negative changes; therefore, access to NR may be necessary at any length of time postinjury. In our experience, the length of time since injury of patients referred to the holistic NR programs that serve the South East of England ranges from 4 weeks to more than 30 years. Most referrals have never received NR before, but some require top-up intervention due to a new problem. The need to access NR in such circumstances is often triggered by movement through the normal developmental stages of life (e.g., changes in living circumstances, work, family, relationships). Therefore, the younger the person is when the index event occurs, the more likely he or she is to need multiple points of access to NR. However, funding of NR internationally does not currently match need or follow the empirical evidence base; instead it is often dictated by resources. For instance, in the United Kingdom, NHS treatment length is capped due to oversubscribed services and under-resourced therapy teams (i.e., insufficient funding); similarly, in the United States, arbitrary restrictions are imposed by medical insurers driven by financial factors rather than the evidence base about recovery rates.

The evidence base regarding the trajectory of recovery has demonstrated that there are several different patterns of recovery to be seen, especially after a TBI (Shiel et al., 2000). The usual pattern is for steady progress until the recovery process plateaus. However, in addition to this group, Shiel et al. identified four other patterns of recovery. First, there is the group who show little evidence of change and remain with a disorder of consciousness (Dewar, Pickard, & Wilson, 2008). The second group consists of the patients who make early rapid progress but plateau quickly. The third group comprises patients who improve rapidly and then make steady progress, while the final group is made up of those who show very little evidence of change for many months before continuing to progress for a long time. See Case Study 1.2, the story of Gary (Wilson et al., 2016) for an example of such a patient. This illustrates how important it is not to make decisions about life and death or withdrawal of treatment too soon. Yet currently, postacute rehabilitation services internationally often limit admissions to 3–6 months.

Over the last 35 years a substantial evidence base has been accumulated internationally that demonstrates early intervention after TBI has positive effects. Just a few of the studies supporting this are listed here (Cope & Hall, 1982; Cowen et al., 1995; Shiel et al., 2001; Greenwood et al., 2004; Satapathy et al., 2016). Most studies have demonstrated decreased overall length of treatment (thus likely delivering cost savings in relation to the overall health economy). It has also been known since 1992 that patients in posttraumatic amnesia (PTA) do have the capacity to learn (Wilson, Baddeley, Evans, & Shiel, 1992), yet despite this there are very few services that provide hyperacute neurorehabilitation to patients with a TBI and/or while the patient is still in PTA. Most patients are left floundering on acute wards waiting for them to naturally emerge from PTA. Unfortunately, as they do, their confusional state results in increased agitation and aggression. It is noteworthy that a 3-year follow-up study of people who had sustained a very severe TBI found that those who had received any kind of rehabilitation were far less likely to exhibit verbal or physical aggression than those who had received no rehabilitation (Shiel, 1999). The economic value of hyperacute rehabilitation for people who are medically unstable with severe physical disability following ABI has been demonstrated (Turner-Stokes et al., 2016) but until recently no studies had looked at the economic impact of delivering such services for the "walking wounded" TBI patients who remain in hyper/acute settings because they are in PTA.

One recent innovative study that looks set to change the way services are commissioned in the United Kingdom for the "walking-wounded" patients with TBI has been described by Dilley and colleagues (2018). They have been running a pilot service for NHS England to evaluate the impact of delivering neuropsychological rehabilitation to the "walking-wounded" survivors of TBI during the hyperacute phase (i.e., while in PTA and requiring acute hospital care for cognitive and behavioral difficulties. Some patients also had severe orthopedic injuries). They compared the results to a matched sample of patients who had received treatment as usual and the preliminary findings are very promising. In the experimental sample there was a statistically significant reduction in the length of days in PTA, the length of rehabilitation required to achieve the same level of recovery as the control group, and the overall length of days spent in the hospital (see Figure 1.1). Collectively, the reduction in bed days demonstrated a substantial financial saving for the NHS and therefore there is strong interest in rolling out this service model nationally in England (NHS England, personal communication, 2018).

More real-world research such as the work of Dilley and colleagues (2018) is required to help facilitate commissioning of services that actually match patient need. We hope that the essential principles of NR as discussed in the following chapters will help inspire clinicians to take up this challenge.

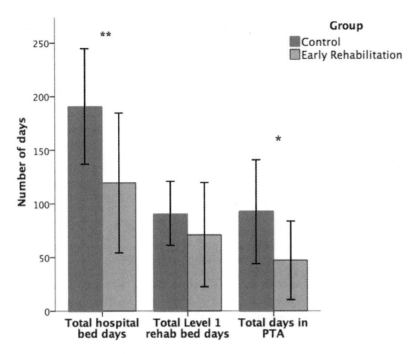

FIGURE 1.1. Outcome of a pilot study delivering hyperacute neuropsychological rehabilitation. *significant as the 0.05 level; **significant at the 0.01 level; error bias 1 = 1 +/–1

Case Study 1.1. Recovery from Hypoxic Brain Injury: The Power of Family Support[1]

Corin Redgrave, the famous actor and playwright, was 65 when he suffered a heart attack while making a speech protesting about the Dale Farm travelers' eviction in 2005.[2] The ambulance reported a downtime of 20 minutes and neuroimaging confirmed severe hypoxic brain injury affecting his hippocampi and frontal end territories. When he emerged from coma he was severely amnesic and confabulating. He

---

[1] See Markham (2014) for an excellent account of the wife's experience of providing support and the complexities involved in this role.

[2] A dispute in which traveling families (a.k.a. Pavees, an itinerant ethnic group of Irish descent) fought a battle with the local governmental body to remain on the land (i.e., Dale Farm), which traveling families had previously been given permission to use. The site had become home to over 1,000 people.

had no insight into his condition and developed severe psychiatric difficulties including aggression and paranoia that necessitated him being detained under the Mental Health Act for his own safety. On discharge he required 24-hour supervision and support to perform basic activities of daily living (ADL) such as washing, dressing, and toileting. He defensively denied that he had any memory impairment and therefore refused to engage in rehabilitation and with carers. As a member of the Redgrave theatrical dynasty, he had an exceptional level of family support and over the course of 2 years he received intensive NR both from the NHS and privately funded neuropsychology sessions. Intervention initially involved spending months working jointly with his wife, Kika, raising his insight and facilitating his acceptance of his cognitive disability via one-on-one neuropsychology sessions.

During this process, Corin identified that his worst fear as an actor had been to lose his memory; he had a premorbid memory of a recurrent nightmare in which he had been about to go on stage but could not recall his lines. He identified his inability to face this fear as the psychological barrier preventing him from engaging in rehabilitation. Once his emotional block was addressed, he began to engage in cognitive rehabilitation; although this was not a linear process and he frequently oscillated between defensively denying his memory impairment and accepting it. Therefore, the process of insight raising and cognitive rehabilitation had to occur simultaneously for several months. Consequently, it took over a year to train him to use a Filofax as a memory aid (see Sohlberg, Johansen, Geyer, & Hoornbeek, 1994). The content of his entries had to include emotionally salient information to help him learn the value of the aid. His whole family (i.e., wife, children, and extended family, especially his sisters) remained heavily involved throughout and received training in how to support him to make entries in the Filofax that would facilitate generalization of skills taught in rehabilitation to everyday life. Their perseverance and determination in partnership with the therapy is what ultimately resulted in him achieving an exceptional outcome. He regained his independence in all activities of daily living and was able to independently mobilize in the community using his compensatory memory aid. He returned to work and completed acting roles using creative compensatory approaches such as having his lines hidden on theater props as a cue. The creativity and support of the theatrical community with the aid of his family's resolve enabled him to supercede all medical expectation. The main message here is that exceptional outcomes can be seen following hypoxic brain injury, but it takes persistence and endurance on the part of both families and therapists to achieve this result. Fundamentally, it is important to note that Corin did not make a good cognitive recovery, he remained severely memory-impaired, but he achieved a good psychological adjustment to his cognitive disability and this enabled him to be less impaired by his cognitive deficits. His family's acceptance of his cognitive deficits and motivation to work with therapists to help him compensate is what resulted in significant gains in relation to his level of functioning and quality of life. The theatrical community's willingess to make adjustments to accommodate his cognitive disabilities is what made his return to work possible. Sadly, not all employers are so accommodating, and therefore vocational restrictions are often due to the inflexibility of the employer rather than the person's cognitive disability.

Case Study 1.2. From Vegetative State to Meaningful Life[3]

In October 2011, Gary, at the age of 28 years, was beaten with metal poles and pieces of wood while protecting his father from a gang of around 30 teenagers. He sustained several fractures to his head, including left orbital and left temporoparietal skull fractures and he developed an acute subdural hematoma. At first, he was awake after a week and was responding to his family. He was then transferred to his local hospital where he fell out of bed, hit his head, and deteriorated. A CT scan showed he had hydrocephalus, so a shunt was inserted to resolve this problem. He later developed seizures and cellulitis over the valve. He was admitted to the Raphael Hospital 4 months later. As he was opening his eyes but not responding to stimuli, he was diagnosed as being in a vegetative state. He was assessed by the neuropsychologist

---

[3] See Wilson, Dhamapurkar, and Rose (2016) for details.

and seen nine times between 4 and 7 months postinjury. He was seen in several different locations, at different times of the day, and with different people present. The locations included Gary's room, physical therapy, and art therapy. He was seen with his mother, other members of his family, the art therapist, two physical therapists, Gary's occupational therapist, and others. Each observation session lasted between 20 and 30 minutes. Gary was usually awake and for the most part quiet during the assessments. He sometimes made a sound (a hiccough or an "oh" sound) and sometimes his left arm would shake. His mother believed this arm shaking was a purposeful movement but no evidence to support this could be found. Gary was reassessed at 11 months postinjury when the report said "No real change." In fact, Gary remained in a vegetative state for nearly 14 months. He then progressed to the minimally conscious state where there was some consistent but limited response to the environment. He was in this state for a further 5 months and was, therefore, deemed to have a disorder of consciousness for 19 months.

With monitored occupational therapy and neuropsychology throughout, Gary emerged from the minimally conscious state and continued to progress for the next 17 months. Treatment included gradual reduction of anti-epileptic drugs, a cranioplasty at 9 months postinjury, occupational therapy, physical therapy, art therapy, music therapy, and other therapeutic interventions. Hydration and nutrients were carefully maintained for the whole of his stay. He left the center walking, talking, with a college application pending, and with above-average scores on some neuropsychological tests. Gary received 3 years rehabilitation (Wilson et al., 2016). He did not emerge from the minimally conscious state until 19 months postinjury. If normal U.K. practice had been followed, he would have been sent to long-term residential care after 6 months or so, and probably would have ended up with contractures and a poor outcome. The main message here is not to stop treating patients too soon.

CHAPTER 2

Who Can Benefit from Neuropsychological Rehabilitation?

Introduction

NR can be implemented by a range of therapists (e.g., neuropsychologists, clinical psychologists, occupational therapists, and speech and language therapists) who work with survivors of ABI. There is a growing body of evidence regarding the value of NR, especially cognitive rehabilitation for people who also have progressive conditions, but it is beyond the scope of this book to meaningfully cover this exciting area of development. Interested readers are encouraged to review the work of John Deluca (2018) and Nadina Lincoln and Avril Drummond for people suffering from multiple sclerosis (Lincoln et al., 2015; Klein et al., 2017). John Deluca's work is of particular significance, as he has demonstrated the effectiveness of cognitive rehabilitation as a group therapy intervention for patients with multiple sclerosis via a randomized controlled trial, and the long-term follow-up data demonstrates maintained generalization of the compensatory skills taught via the group into clients' everyday life (Deluca, 2018). For further information about cognitive rehabilitation with people suffering from dementia, please refer to the seminal work of Linda Clare (Clare et al., 2013), especially the multicenter G.R.E.A.T. study (Goal-oriented cognitive Rehabilitation in Early-stage Alzheimer's and related dementias single-blind randomized controlled Trial), which is funded by the U.K.

Health Technology Assessment Programme and is certain to define the future of dementia care. Morris (2018) provides 10 useful benchmark questions that practitioners working with people with dementia should ask themselves. We suggest these questions should also apply to all practitioners working in NR. The questions apply to all our clients. These questions are:

1. Is the approach advocating individualized care, taking into account the person's individual needs?
2. Is the approach person-centered taking account of the dementia journey and the person's identity?
3. Does the approach involve listening to people with dementia and ensuring their voice is heard?
4. Does the approach advocate involving the person with dementia in decision making regarding their care?
5. Does the approach advocate support for the person with dementia to exercise choices and control?
6. Does the approach advocate and facilitate access to meaningful activities?
7. Does the approach promote participation in local communities that are dementia-friendly?
8. Is the approach focused on enabling the persons to live lives that are meaningful and satisfying?
9. Does the approach consider the impact on the stigma of dementia?
10. Does the approach promote social inclusion and involvement in valued roles and activities?

Main Diagnostic Groups Seen in Rehabilitation

This chapter describes the four main diagnostic groups that have been found to benefit from NR: *TBI, stroke, encephalitis,* and *hypoxia.* However, it is important to emphasize that in clinical practice the diagnosis is less important than the manifestation of problems experienced in everyday life, as tackling the latter is the main purpose of NR. Despite differences in activities and approach among the various professions who implement NR, they each deal with similar problems exhibited by the people with whom they work, including those with motor- and sensory-functioning impairments, cognitive deficits, emotional difficulties, behavioral problems, poor social skills, pain, and fatigue. After considering the work of each of the diagnostic groups, this chapter concludes with a brief description of the main difficulties shared by all groups.

Traumatic Brain Injury

TBI can be defined as an "alteration in brain function, or other evidence of brain pathology, caused by an external force" (Menon, Schwab, Wright, & Maas, 2010, p. 1637). The two main types of TBI are closed head injury and penetrating wounds. Closed head injury (CHI) is by far the most common, accounting for some 70% of TBIs (Ponsford, 2013). It is associated with acceleration and deceleration forces that may or may not involve skull fracture. Severity of brain injury is usually judged by (1) the depth and duration of coma, and (2) the length of posttraumatic amnesia (PTA). Coma can be defined as "a state of unrousable unresponsiveness, lasting more than 6 hours, in which a person cannot be awakened; fails to respond normally to painful stimuli, light or sound; lacks a normal sleep–wake cycle; *and* does not initiate voluntary actions" (Royal College of Physicians, 2013). PTA has been described as "a period of variable length following closed head trauma during which the patient is confused, disorientated, suffers from retrograde amnesia, and seems to lack the capacity to store and retrieve new information" (Schacter & Crovitz, 1977). Even though an old definition, this is still very accurate.

Throughout the world, the most widely used measure of the depth and duration of coma is the Glasgow Coma Scale (GCS; Teasdale & Jennett, 1974). The GCS consists of three sections: eye-opening, verbal, and motor responses. The original 14-point scale of the GCS, later extended to 15 points, provides an uncomplicated and objective measure of coma that is easy to score. Within each section the best possible response is scored 4, 5, or 6, depending on the component being measured and the version of the test employed. The worst possible score for each section is 1; thus even patients who are brain dead score 3.

There are three generally acknowledged levels of severity of TBI, which are based on the Mayo Classification System for Traumatic Brain Injury Severity (Malec, 2004): mild, moderate, and severe. Mild TBI involves a trauma to the head resulting in a confused state or a loss of consciousness of less than 30 minutes, an initial GCS score of 13–15, and PTA lasting less than 24 hours. Moderate TBI involves a trauma to the head resulting in a loss of consciousness between 30 minutes to 24 hours, an initial GCS score of 9–12, and a PTA lasting 24 hours–7 days. Severe TBI results from a trauma to the head leading to a loss of consciousness greater than 24 hours, an initial GCS score of 3–8, and a PTA period of greater than 7 days.

Although the depth and duration of coma is a predictor of long-term outcome, PTA is believed to be an even better predictor (Nakase-Richardson et al., 2011). Jennett (1990) classifies PTA of less than 5 minutes as a very mild head injury, 5–60 minutes as mild, 1-14 hours as moderate, 1–7 days as severe, 1–4 weeks as very severe, and more than 4 weeks as extremely severe. Although he says, "there is no need to seek a very accurate figure for PTA; what matters is whether it lasted minutes, hours, days or weeks" (p. 4).

Ponsford and Dymowski (2017) state that motor vehicle accidents, falls, assaults, bicycle accidents, and sporting injuries are the most common causes of TBI, and the incidence tends to be greatest in young children, older adolescents, and elderly people. There is a gender difference too, with men being one and a half to three times more likely to sustain a TBI than women. Approximately 20% of TBIs result in moderate-to-severe brain damage with the remainder sustaining mild damage (Bruns & Hauser, 2003).

Another factor to be born in mind with regard to survivors of TBI is that the damage caused can be due to primary or to secondary reasons. Primary damage results directly from the accident or assault, whereas secondary damage is due to complications arising from the first insult (Nudo, 2013). Secondary damage may result in a host of complications including cerebral swelling, low blood pressure, infections, and hydrocephalus.

Once an accident has occurred, the primary damage is there and has to be managed as well as possible with the resources available. The secondary damage, however, which sometimes results in more permanent and more severe disability than the primary damage, is (at least potentially) preventable (Teasdale & Mendelow, 1984). For further discussion, see Wilson (2017) and Ponsford and Dymowski (2017). The resulting complications faced by survivors of TBI will be covered later in the chapter.

Stroke

Cerebrovascular accident (CVA) or stroke can be caused by a number of different pathologies including a blocked artery, a leaking or burst blood vessel, or the result of certain conditions such as sickle cell disease or diabetes. The common factor is a sudden onset of focal cerebral damage. Risk of stroke can be reduced by life style changes including stopping smoking, reducing alcohol intake, taking regular exercise, eating a healthy diet, and maintaining a healthy life style. By far the most common type of stroke, about 85% of all strokes, results from ischemia, which is a blockage of the arteries (Stroke Association, 2017: www.stroke.org.uk). About half of ischemic strokes are due to atherosclerosis: this is the term used for hardening and thickening of the arteries. Other causes include (1) cerebral thrombosis where a blood clot formed in one of the arteries leading to the brain becomes blocked; (2) an embolism (a blood clot or piece of fatty tissue from elsewhere in the body) is carried to the brain via the bloodstream; (3) small vessel disease where small blood vessels deep in the brain become blocked causing a stroke, which are sometimes called lacunar strokes; and (4) other rarer causes of ischemic stroke such as a tear in the wall of an artery or to certain heart conditions (Stroke Association, 2017). The remaining 15% or so of strokes are due to cerebral hemorrhage, that is bleeding into the brain, and these are more likely to affect older people. Although most hemorrhagic strokes are within the brain itself, a significant minority are due to a sub-arachnoid hemorrhage (SAH), which is caused by bleeding into the lining of the brain. About 25% of patients with stroke are below the age of 65 and many of these will have sustained a subarachnoid hemorrhage. Although only 5–10% of strokes are caused by a SAH, they are important because they tend to affect a younger age group (Mayo Clinic, 2017). Most, between 50 and 80% of SAHs, are caused by a ruptured aneurysm (similar to a bubble on an artery); however, a few are due to an angioma, which is an abnormal blood vessel. Women have a slightly higher risk than men; and the average age is 50 years (Mayo Clinic, 2017). Most aneurysms occur in the forks of arteries and some sites are more affected than others, with the anterior communi-cating artery frequently affected. Survivors of a SAH are often seen in brain injury rehabilitation centers.

In the United Kingdom approximately 150,000 people have a stroke each year (Stroke Association, 2017). It is not only the third most common cause of death but also the leading cause of severe dis-ability; and more than 250,000 people live with disabilities caused by stroke in the United Kingdom. Mozaffarian et al. (2016) provide fig-ures for the United States. They report that every year some 795,000 people have a new or recurrent stroke (ischemic or hemorrhagic) and one in every 20 deaths in the United States is due to a stroke, with someone dying every 4 minutes. Van Heugten (2017a) reports that worldwide about 15 million people a year sustain a stroke of whom 5 million die and 5 million are permanently disabled. It is worth men-tioning here that some people experience a mini- or temporary stroke called a transient ischemic attack (TIA), which lasts no longer than 24 hours. Despite its brevity, the Stroke Association warns that TIAs are serious and considered to be warning strokes.

As with other kinds of brain damage, the consequences of stroke are many and include motor, sensory, cognitive, emotional, and behav-ioral problems. Treatment of these will be covered later in the book.

For a thorough coverage of the psychological management of stroke survivors, see Lincoln, Kneebone, Macniven, and Morris (2012).

Encephalitis

Encephalitis refers to an inflammation of the brain (Granerod & Crowcroft, 2007). Despite its low rate of occurrence, its effects can have variable and sometimes extreme consequences. There are two major types of encephalitis: the first is caused by an infection from a virus, bacteria, or parasite; the second results from an abnormal immune response in which the body attacks itself (Stone & Hawkins, 2007). Autoimmune responses can be triggered by a recent infection or vaccination. The most common infections, at least in the Western world, are those caused by the herpes simplex virus (the same virus that causes the common cold sore) and varicella zoster (the virus that causes chicken pox and shingles). Measles, mumps, and cytomegalavirus are some of the other viruses that can cause inflammation of the brain. In other parts of the world, West Nile virus, Japanese virus, and viruses from bites of ticks or mosquitos may be the cause (Stone & Hawkins, 2007; Stapley, Atkins, & Easton, 2009). However, in more than 50% of cases, the infecting virus cannot be determined (Stapley et al., 2009; Granerod & Crowcroft, 2007). Easton and Hodgson (2017) point out that in some cases where patients are immune-compromised or where the cause cannot be identified, encephalitis can present in a slow and chronic form that may ultimately lead to death.

Of the noninfectious encephalopathies, the inflammation of the brain is caused by the central nervous system attacking itself. Acute disseminated encephalomyelitis (ADEM) is an acute demyelinating condition mainly affecting children and young adults. One study showed that it was triggered by an infectious illness or vaccination in 74% of cases (Stone & Hawkins, 2007). For an account of a young woman with ADEM, see Kate's Story (in Wilson & Bainbridge, 2014).

There are, of course, other kinds of auto-immune encephalopathies. One relatively rare form of auto-immune encephalitis is anti-NMDA (N-methyl-D-aspartate) receptor encephalitis. Although this is an acute and potentially lethal type of the illness caused by an auto-immune reaction, it is also one that has a high probability of recovery. An excellent book, written by a survivor of this form of encephalitis is Cahalan (2012). As described in Wilson, Robertson, and Mole (2015), Susannah Cahalan was a successful young reporter for the *New York Post* when she started to become unwell with strange symptoms at the age of 24. Following significant deterioration and experiencing hallucinations, paranoia, and seizures, she received several incorrect diagnoses from the medical profession. One said she had a breakdown caused by stress and another explained her symptoms as problems with withdrawal due to alcoholism. Both these explanations turned out to be totally untrue. She became extremely thin, was hospitalized, and came close to being admitted to a long-stay psychiatric unit. One undertaking she did not experience at this time was a neuropsychological assessment, which would have probably diagnosed an organic deficit much sooner. Eventually, Susannah was seen by a psychiatrist, Dr. Najjar, who gave her the classic "clock" test (usually administered by a neuropsychologist). This showed that she had unilateral neglect (most often associated with right hemisphere stroke) caused by an organic rather than an emotional problem. A biopsy followed, revealing that her brain was inflamed: cells from her immune system had attacked nerve cells in her brain. Having only been identified 4 years before she became ill, Susannah Cahalan was the 217th person in the world to be diagnosed with this rare disorder. Treatment began and she slowly improved, was able to return to work, and continues to be a brilliant journalist as well as a gifted speaker.

Encephalitis typically begins with an influenza-type illness or headache followed, hours or days later, by more serious symptoms, which can include a drop in the level of consciousness, high temperature, seizures, sensitivity to light, and other changes in behavior. The types of symptoms seen in encephalitis reflect the specific areas of the brain affected by inflammation (Stapley et al., 2009). The illness is difficult to diagnose due to the range of possible symptoms and the wide variety in the rate of development.

Granerod et al. (2013) believe that the incidence of encephalitis is higher than previously thought. The only study looking at the incidence in the United Kingdom at that time (Davison et al., 2003) reported 1.5 cases per 100,000 population per year for viral encephalitis alone. However, as most cases are of unknown etiology and there are an increasing number of viruses known to cause the condition, this was felt to be a serious underestimate. Furthermore, many cases are not reported despite the fact that encephalitis is a notifiable disease in the United Kingdom.

Following on from these observations, Granerod and her colleagues (2013) carried out a thorough investigation of hospital records to estimate the number of encephalitis cases in England "attributable to infectious and noninfectious causes" (2013, p. 1455). They found an incidence rate of 5.23 cases per 100,000 population per year. The incidence rate was highest among patients below 1 year and over 65 years of age. Females were 8% less likely to contract the disease than males. Compared to other infectious diseases, encephalitis has a high mortality rate. Some 10% of those with encephalitis die from their infections or complications resulting from secondary infection. Some forms of encephalitis have more severe outcomes including herpes encephalitis, in which mortality is 15–20% with treatment and 70–80% without treatment (Stapley et al., 2009).

Two recent books provide detailed accounts of people with the condition. Wilson et al., (2015) is cowritten by Claire, a survivor of herpes simplex viral encephalitis, which left her with a very severe prosopagnosia and loss of people knowledge. The other book, by Ava Easton (2016), chief executive officer of the Encephalitis Society, provides an account of people with encephalitis and its consequences for them and their families. Help for survivors and their families, as well as for those who have lost a loved one is provided by the Encephalitis Society (www.encephalitis.info).

Hypoxia

Hypoxia simply means reduced oxygen to the body's tissues while anoxia refers to lack of oxygen to these tissues. The terms are often used interchangeably. Hypoxic brain damage happens when insufficient oxygen has reached the brain, causing it to cease to function adequately. All tissues of the human body require oxygen in order to perform properly. The brain, however, needs more oxygen than other organs. Weighing approximately 2% of an adult's entire weight, the brain uses about 20% of the energy produced. Lack of this energy in the form of oxygen can result in permanent brain damage. As Hossman (1999) stated, "The high energy requirements compared to the low energy reserves render the brain particularly vulnerable to hypoxic conditions" (p. 155). A diminished supply of oxygen before, during, or shortly after birth may lead to developmental delays. Those who suffer hypoxic damage after this period, however, are more likely to have sustained a cardiac or pulmonary arrest or an embolism, or else they have attempted suicide (particularly with carbon monoxide poisoning); taken a drug overdose; survived hanging, drowning, or an anesthetic accident; or have experienced oxygen deprivation as a result of stroke or traumatic brain injury. Wilson and van Heugten (2017) describe this result in more detail. Attempted suicide with carbon monoxide poisoning is, perhaps, the most common cause of hypoxic brain injury seen in adult rehabilitation centers together with hypoxia associated with TBI. Although cardiac arrests are common, these are often seen in older people who are not referred to brain injury rehabilitation centers.

While the rate at which different areas of the brain become damaged following shortage of oxygen varies widely, the areas most at risk are the "watershed" regions of the cortex. This is because the vascular supply is dependent on the furthest radiations of the cerebral arteries (Wilson & van Heugten, 2017). The areas involved in autonomic functions are most resistant to shortage of oxygen. The basal ganglia are another area susceptible to hypoxia (Caine & Watson, 2000). Hossman (1999) offers a different point of view, which indicates that the brain regions most sensitive to this type of injury are parts of the hippocampus, the dorsolateral caudate nucleus, and the reticular nucleus of the thalamus.

Wilson and van Heugten (2017) note that cognitive and emotional problems are common after hypoxic brain damage. Caregivers may also experience a high burden and they often have emotional problems, including symptoms of posttraumatic stress disorder (PTSD). Of the various cognitive deficits that are observed, depending on the extent and severity of brain damage, memory and executive disorders are the most typical. Wilson (1996a) noted that 33% of 18 patients had both memory and executive problems as their major cognitive deficits, while Caine and Watson (2000) found 54% of 67 patients had a memory disorder. Peskine, Picq, and Pradat-Diehl (2004) recognized executive problems in all 12 of their anoxic patients. The pure amnesic syndrome is also seen, although less often (only 13 or 19.4% in the Caine and Watson review and only three or nearly 17% in the Wilson sample). Visuospatial and visuoperceptual deficits may result too. Wilson (1996a) found two patients had these problems in addition to their memory and executive difficulties, with another three patients having visualperceptual and visualspatial problems alone. Caine and Watson (2000) found 21 cases (31.3%) with these difficulties. Disorders of recognition such as visual object agnosia and Balint's syndrome, of which the most striking deficit involves problems localizing in space, are rare but when they are seen they nearly always result from anoxic or hypoxic brain damage (Wilson et al., 2005; Wilson, Evans, Gracey, & Bateman, 2009).

Some survivors of hypoxia have such severe impairment that they cannot be assessed with traditional neuropsychological tests and have to be assessed with tests for people with special needs. Such a group comprised almost 25% of the Wilson (1996a) sample. Finally, there are those who remain with a disorder of consciousness (DOC) who are in a vegetative state (VS) or a minimally conscious state (MCS). Giacino and Whyte (2005) recognized that patients who are in a VS or an MCS following anoxic damage do less well than those whose DOC follows a TBI. In 2015, Dhamapurkar, Wilson, Rose, and Florschutz (2015) et al. found that 18% of 28 people who had a DOC for 12 or more months recovered consciousness and that survivors of a TBI were more likely to show delayed recovery than non-TBI patients, most of whom had sustained hypoxic brain damage. These were less likely to recover. In short, the problems seen in survivors of hypoxic brain damage are no different from those seen in survivors of other kinds of nonprogressive brain damage including TBI, stroke, and encephalitis.

Problems Faced by Survivors of Nonprogressive Brain Injury

As stated several times in this chapter, the difficulties faced by all people with nonprogressive brain injury are similar, whatever the cause of their brain injury. Most people receiving rehabilitation for the consequences of brain injury have both cognitive and noncognitive problems. A typical patient in a rehabilitation center will have several cognitive problems such as poor attention, memory, planning, and organizational difficulties together with some emotional problems such as anxiety, depression, or in some cases PTSD. The patient may exhibit behavior problems such as poor self-control or anger outbursts; there may be some subtle motor difficulties leading to reduced stamina and unsteady gait; there may well be problems connected with social skills and relationships; family members probably do not understand what has happened to the person they once felt they knew and understood; and there will probably be issues connected with the continuation of work or education. These are the difficulties we have to deal with in rehabilitation and will address later in this book.

Rehabilitation Around the World: Similarities, Struggles, and Solutions

Western countries such as the United States and the United Kingdom can learn from countries with limited resources. Indeed, we all face similar difficulties. For example, there are too few trained staff, too many people needing help, language and cultural issues, and questions as to how far to engage families in the rehabilitation process. On the one hand, families are not trained professional staff and as we will see with EO in Chapter 6, wives want to be wives not caretakers. On the other hand, families are with patients more often, they know patients better than anyone, and, where rehabilitation services are lacking, engaging the help of families may be the only realistic option. Training family members is best summed up by Shah (2017) when she explains that in India there are few trained professionals and rehabilitation centers, minimal interdisciplinary coordination, and no government funding or private insurance for rehabilitation services, but there are large, supportive family units with a culture of living together and interdependence. This has resulted in a trend of training family members, with professionals becoming consultants rather than primary service providers. Single therapists often have to manage the case and offer guidance about all aspects of rehabilitation. Individual therapy for cognitive, emotional, and psychosocial problems is not feasible, so group sessions replace individual ones. The strength of this family-centric, transdisciplinary model is that the focus shifts to functional recovery that is relevant and of value to the individual. All this can be and is sometimes done in the United States, the United Kingdom, and other Western countries. However, warns Shah, inadequate skills, caregiver burnout, overprotection, or overzealous management by family members are concerns.

In a recent international handbook (Wilson, Winegardner, van Geugten, & Ownsworth, 2017), people from 10 different countries described their perception of rehabilitation in their own lands. These ranged from countries with very large populations such as China and India to those with very small populations. Botswana, for example, has only 2 million people. Another difference was by the number of languages spoken in a country. Only one language dominates in Brazil, Argentina, and Iran, while there are 11 official languages in South Africa and an even greater number in India, where there appears to be no agreement on just how many languages are spoken. In multicultural countries such as the United States and the United Kingdom, we may not have so many official languages but most neuropsychologists face situations where an interpreter is needed and the cultural systems of clients are different from those of the person carrying out the assessment. Funding issues are a challenge wherever we live and work. Many rehabilitation programs in the United Kingdom are funded by the NHS and this often pays for people in private centers if nowhere else can be found for them to go. In the United States most treatment is paid for by insurance claims but this focuses on acute and early postacute care or else nursing home care; and the kind of rehabilitation lasting several months is less often paid for except in places where the state funds vocational rehabilitation. This is not, of course, the whole picture and there is variability based on the particular insurance plan and the predetermined benefits patients have signed up for. Sometimes benefits continue longer than a few weeks, based on demonstrated progress. Also, some insurance programs fund medically necessary therapies to improve home independence (Pamela Klonoff, personal communication, 2018).

Hopefully, all countries recognize that rehabilitation is not synonymous with recovery if by "recovery" it is meant getting back to what one was like before injury or illness; and all accept that rehabilitation is not synonymous with treatment as the latter is something we *do to* people or *give to* them, whereas rehabilitation is a two-way interactive process. As we said earlier, NR is concerned with the amelioration of cognitive, emotional, psychosocial, and behavioral deficits caused by an insult to the brain. Its main purpose is to enable people with disabilities to achieve their optimum level of well-being, to reduce the impact of their problems in everyday life, and to help them return to their own most appropriate environments. Its purpose is not to teach individuals to score better on tests or to learn lists of words or to be faster at detecting stimuli. However much countries differ, the definition and purpose of rehabilitation is something all can agree on.

Finally, in this chapter we would like to remind readers that this book is for people in all countries and not solely for the more developed ones. We have much to learn from each other.

CHAPTER 3

The Purposes and Process of Neuropsychological Rehabilitation

Introduction

Rehabilitation should enable people with disabilities to achieve their optimum level of well-being, to reduce the impact of difficulties experienced in everyday life, and to help them return to their own most appropriate environments. While the collection of data from tests during rehabilitation has its place in analyzing problems experienced by individuals, helping them to score better on tests or learn lists of words or detect stimuli are not targets in themselves. Data from standardized tests help us build up a picture of a person's strengths and weaknesses, while data from observations and other behavioral assessments can answer questions about real-life problems. We look at these points in more detail later in Chapter 5. In NR, as far as possible, one needs to address real-life difficulties experienced by people with brain injuries unless one is asking a particular question that cannot be answered in this way. The results, however, should then be applicable to real-life issues.

Practical Implications of Research

An example of how research within the field of rehabilitation might proceed, given the above strictures, is the following from Baddeley and Wilson (1994) and Wilson, Baddeley, Evans, and Shiel (1994). They first asked the question "Do people with amnesia learn more if prevented from making mistakes while learning?" This was answered with an experiment whereby three groups of participants, young people, older people, and people with severe amnesia, were given lists of words in two conditions. In one of them participants were compelled to make errors and in the second condition they were prevented from making errors. Conditions were counterbalanced. Every one of the people with severe amnesia learned more when errors were prevented. As articulated above, rehabilitation is not about teaching people lists of words, so the next step was to see if preventing errors also led to better learning in everyday life. A series of single-case experimental designs showed this was the case and since then errorless learning has been a mainstay in memory rehabilitation (Wilson, 2009).

The Starting Point in the Rehabilitation Process

In any rehabilitation program, the starting point is the person with neuropsychological problems together with his or her family. We should find out what his or her needs are, what he or she wants to achieve, and what is preventing him or her from coping with the demands of everyday life. Preinjury coping styles, mental health, social and ethnic background, and lifestyle of the person with brain injury (and other family members) will impact on the needs and desires of these people and thus on the rehabilitation offered. The nature, extent, and severity of the brain damage need to be determined. This may well be obtained through hospital notes and brain imaging. We also need to interview the patient, the family, and other concerned individuals. It is, of course, necessary to identify current cognitive, emotional, psychosocial, and behavioral problems; and models of language, reading, memory, executive functioning, attention, and perception are all available to provide detailed information about an individual's attributes and deficits. Assessment procedures for emotional, behavioral, and social issues, emanating from theories of coping, adjustment, social and personal identity, attachment theory, systemic theories, and others, can be employed. Behavioral or functional assessments will complement standardized assessment procedures (Wilson, Winegardner, & Ashworth, 2014). These are addressed in Chapter 5, which deals with assessment. Having identified problems, it will be necessary to decide on appropriate rehabilitation strategies, involving the negotiation of suitable goals that are meaningful and functionally relevant. The person with brain injury, family members, and rehabilitation staff should all be involved in the negotiating process. Although there may be times or stages in the recovery process where it is appropriate to focus on impairments, the majority of goals for those engaged in NR will address disabilities that impact on activities and handicaps that limit participation in society (World Health Organization, 2001). Goal setting in rehabilitation is addressed in more detail in Chapters 7 and 8.

Can We Restore Lost Functioning?

There is obviously more than one way to try to achieve any goal. Should we try to restore lost functioning, encourage anatomical reorganization, help people use their residual skills more efficiently, find an alternative means to the final goal through compensations (functional adaptation), use environmental modifications to bypass problems, or use a combination of these methods?

Whether or not it is possible to restore lost functioning is a debatable point and this may depend on the cognitive function itself. While there is no evidence, for example, that memory functioning can be restored in someone with the amnesic syndrome (Wilson, 2009), it is less clear whether we might be able to restore other functions such as attention or language (Evans, 2009; Raymer & Turkstra, 2017). Sometimes we can improve people's attention skills through retraining, but these improvements tend not to generalize to real-life tasks (Fish, 2017). In addition, there may be disagreement as to whether change is due to restoration or to compensation. Take problem solving as an example. There is evidence that problem-solving training leads to improved problem solving (Levine et al., 2000; Evans, 2009), yet it is not clear whether this means problem-solving *ability* has been improved or whether people with problem-solving difficulties have been given a compensatory strategy with which to deal with their problems.

Can an Undamaged Part of the Brain Take Over the Functions of a Damaged Part?

Another approach that is sometimes considered possible is to enable an undamaged part of the brain to take over the function of a damaged part. This is what is meant by *anatomical reorganization*. Although we know this can happen in babies and infants (Kohn & Dennis, 1978), it is often at the expense of other functions (Dennis & Kohn,1975); and it is less clear to what extent this might happen in adults. Some anatomical reorganization does occur in some circumstances, as we know from the studies of taxi drivers (Maguire et al., 2000) when MRI scans were taken of the brains of taxi drivers with extensive knowledge of London routes and compared with non-taxi drivers. The posterior hippocampi of taxi drivers were significantly larger than those of people who were not taxi drivers and the difference in size correlated with the amount of time spent as a taxi driver. Van Heugten (2017b) reports on a few other studies demonstrating increase in various brain regions in the adult human brain following extensive practice. Nevertheless, it is unclear as to what extent this can be used as a treatment strategy in brain injury rehabilitation. We do know that some amnesic patients have had extensive practice in memory exercises with no change in everyday memory performance (Wilson, 1999). Once again, it may be the type of cognitive function that determines improvement.

Robertson and Murre (1999) believe that two mechanisms can cause plastic reorganization. The first is due to a rapidly occurring alteration in synaptic activity taking place over seconds or minutes, while the second is because of structural changes taking place over days and weeks. The authors suggest that some people show spontaneous recovery with no specific intervention; others, however, show very little recovery, even over a period of years. Compensatory approaches should be used with this latter group. Others show reasonably good recovery provided they receive rehabilitation, and these are described as the assisted recovery group with whom issues of plasticity can be addressed. It is also believed by Robertson and Murre that the severity of brain damage determines which group people belong to. Thus, mild lesions result in spontaneous recovery; people with moderate lesions benefit from assisted recovery; and those with severe lesions require the compensatory approach.

As we said in Chapter 1, although there may be some truth in this concept of differing severity, it is probably limited in comparison with the actual location of the lesion, which almost certainly plays a crucial role in rehabilitation. For example, people with mild lesions in the frontal lobes could be more disadvantaged in terms of responding to rehabilitation than people with severe lesions in the hippocampus. The former group might have attention, planning, and organization difficulties precluding them from gaining the maximum benefit from the rehabilitation offered, whereas the latter group, with memory problems, could compensate well (Wilson, 2009). Once again, however, we stress that all those who do not show spontaneous recovery require rehabilitation.

Teaching People to Use Their Residual Skills More Efficiently

One of the most important types of strategy used in NR is teaching people to use their residual skills more efficiently. In this approach, it is assumed that some residual functioning remains. For example, people with amnesia do not lose *all* memory functioning and can possibly be helped to use what little remains more effectively. This might include allowing extra time to learn new information and making associations between the new information they are trying to remember and the old information they already know. Mnemonics probably work because they allow previously isolated items to become integrated with one another (Bower, 1972). Many of the memory therapy techniques described by Wilson (2009) follow this approach. Rehearsal techniques such as Landauer and Bjork's (1978) method of expanding rehearsal (otherwise known as spaced retrieval) have been employed with people with dementia (Camp, Bird, & Cherry, 2000; Clare, 2008) and by people with TBI (Wilson, 2009). This method involves the presentation of material to be remembered (e.g., a new name or telephone number) followed by immediate testing and then a gradual building up of the retention interval. In these studies people were helped to use their residual skills more efficiently.

This strategy does not apply solely to those with memory difficulties: people with executive deficits, for example, do not lose *all* their ability to plan, organize, or problem solve and many of the rehabilitation programs encourage this group to use the abilities they have more efficiently. Goal management training (Levine et al., 2000) is a method whereby a "goal management framework" (GMF) is introduced to enable people to enhance their problem-solving abilities. Based on the work of Duncan (1986) and Robertson (1996), the GMF is a six-step problem-solving strategy:

1. Stop and think! What am I doing? Check the mental blackboard.
2. Define the main task.
3. List the step-solving difficulties that are provided with this framework, usually printed on a little laminated card that can be kept in a pocket and referred to when needed.
4. Learn these steps.
5. Do it.
6. Am I doing what I planned?

They are given practice in following through the steps, at first with hypothetical problems and then with real-life problems. Some people internalize the steps, while others will require the GMF as a permanent *aide-mémoire* (see Winegardner, 2017, for further details on how this is implemented in clinical practice).

Compensation

A crucial procedure in the rehabilitation of neuropsychological deficits is enabling people to *compensate* for their problems, particularly those that are considered to be cognitive. However, emotional problems can also be included. This is part of the functional adaptation or *finding an alternative means to the final goal* approach. Computers can, for example, be used as cognitive prosthetics, as compensatory devices, as assessment tools, or as a means for training. Given the current expansion in information technology, this is likely to be an area of growth and increasing importance in the next decade. One of the earliest papers describing the use of an electronic aid with a person with brain damage was Kurlychek (1983), who showed that a real-life problem, in this case involving the checking of a timetable, could be overcome. In 1986, Glisky and Schacter taught memory-impaired people computer terminology, and one of their participants was able to find employment as a computer operator. Kirsch and his colleagues (Kirsch, Levine, Fallon-Krueger, & Jaros, 1987) designed an interactive task guidance system to assist brain-injured people perform everyday tasks. Boake (2003) includes discussion of some of the early computer-based programs. Since then, there have been numerous papers reporting successful use of technology with brain-injured people. Wilson, Emslie, Quirk, and Evans (2001) used a randomized controlled crossover design to demonstrate that it is possible to reduce the everyday problems of neurologically impaired people with memory and/or planning problems. Another area where technology is likely to play an increasing role in the future is virtual reality (VR). VR can be used to simulate real-life situations and thus can be beneficial for both assessment and treatment (Rose, Brooks, & Rizzo, 2005). For an up-to-date review, see O'Neill, Jamieson, and Goodwin (2017) who provide a fascinating account of the way assistive technology can be used to help those with disorders of attention, memory, and emotion; higher-level cognitive functions; calculation; self and time functions; recognition of objects, actions, and faces; and everyday life navigation.

Environmental Modifications

The final strategy that is employed in NR is modifying or adapting the environment in order to reduce cognitive demands (e.g., painting the bathroom doors a distinctive color so they can be easily distinguished from other doors or working in a quiet, nondistracting room to aid concentration). This intervention is particularly useful for those with severe and widespread cognitive difficulties. Just as those with severe physical disabilities can cope in a modified environment so can those with severe cognitive problems. Take, for example, people who are totally paralyzed from the neck down. With the appropriate equipment they can control their physical environments through a voice-activated control device or by using their mouths to control a stick. Through these mechanisms they can open and close doors and windows, turn the pages of a book, answer the telephone, and so forth. The disabled person controls the structured environment through his or her mouth and no longer needs the use of limbs to do this. Similarly, a person with severe cognitive impairments can be enabled to function in a suitably structured environment with signposts, labeling of doors, reminders from staff, and alarms that alert caregivers if the person wanders off. "Smart houses" for people with cognitive deficits have been designed (Gartland, 2004) in an attempt to "disable the disabling environment." These environments are controlled by computers, video links, and telephones, and they can remind people about toilets, baths, and medication; ensure that showers are the right temperature; and turn electrical appliances on and off.

Kapur, Glisky, and Wilson (2004) indicate that environmental aids can be subdivided into proximal and distal aids. The proximal environment covers the design and contents of a room or vehicle and the equipment an individual uses in everyday settings. In his wonderful book *The Psychology of Everyday Things,* Norman (1988) argues that knowledge should be in the world rather than in the head. By this he means that if we approach a door it should be obvious whether or not we should push or pull to open it. If we are using a stove it should be obvious which knob controls which burner. We should not have to remember these things, as the design should make it obvious. This is the same principle behind the concept of environmental aids in NR.

Thus, someone with severe executive deficits may be able to function in a structured environment, with no distractions and where there is no need to problem solve, as the task at hand is clear and unambiguous. Similarly, people with severe memory problems may not be handicapped in environments where there are no demands made on memory. Thus, if doors, cupboards, drawers, and storage jars are clearly labeled, if rooms are cleared of dangerous equipment, if someone appears to remind or accompany the memory-impaired person when it is time to go to the dentist or to eat dinner, the affected person may cope reasonably well.

Kapur et al. (2004) give other examples. Items can be left by the front door for people who forget to take belongings with them when they leave the house; a message can be left on the mirror in the hallway; and a simple flow chart can be used to help people search in likely places when they cannot find a lost belonging (Moffat, 1989). Cars, mobile phones, and other items may have intrinsic alarms to remind people to do things. These can be paired with voice messages to remind people why the alarm is ringing. Modifications can also be made to verbal environments to avoid irritating behavior such as the repetition of a question, story, or joke. It might be possible to identify a "trigger" or an antecedent that elicits this behavior. Thus, by eliminating the "trigger" one can avoid the repetitious behavior. For example, in response to the question "How are you today?", one young man who had survived a traumatic brain injury would always say "Just getting over my hangover." Amusing at first, this response soon becomes irritating. If staff simply said "Good morning," however, he replied "Good morning," so the repetitive comments about his supposed hangover were avoided. Proximal environmental aids therefore involve structuring the immediate environment and organizing the equipment or material in the environment to reduce the load on a person's cognitive functioning.

Distal environmental aids, on the other hand, involve the wider environment and include the layout of buildings, shopping centers, streets and towns, office buildings, hospitals, and residential homes. These can differ in their effectiveness in helping people get around. In some the sign posting, color coding, alarm systems, and warning signs are excellent in reducing the chances of getting lost or falling downstairs, and others should be improved to reach similar standards, thereby reducing cognitive load in ways in which proximal environmental aids have succeeded.

In practice, we use a combination of approaches in NR. The Wilson, Rous, and Sopena (2008) study, which asked practicing neuropsychologists how they went about their professional work in NR, found that all respondents endorsed the use of three approaches: namely, helping people use their residual skills more efficiently, finding an alternative means to the final goal (compensations), and modifying the environment. Only a third, however, said they tried to restore lost functioning or attempted anatomical reorganization.

Whichever method is selected, one should be aware of theories of learning. In Baddeley's words, "A theory of rehabilitation without a model of learning is a vehicle without an engine" (Baddeley, 1993 p. 235). Given contemporary ideas about the interplay between social, emotional, and cognitive functioning, one might also call upon models of therapeutic change to help understand the interpersonal conditions, such as therapeutic working alliance, or the client's experience of being understood, that optimize learning and engagement in rehabilitation. The "Y-shaped" model of the rehabilitation process (Gracey, Evans, & Malley, 2009) suggests that the *plan–do–reflect* cycle, as used to support experiential learning in CBT (see Bennett-Levy et al., 2004) can be used so that even if someone chooses inappropriate goals due to poor awareness, conducting an "experiment" to test out his or her perspective, if done well, can help the person or family "update" their stand point. Often the psychologist's or therapist's perspective is updated too. Recent theories of identity are also proving useful in rehabilitation (Ownsworth, 2014).

The final question is, how best to evaluate success or failure? Consider Whyte's (1997) view that outcome should be congruent with the level of intervention. If intervening at the impairment (body structure and process) level, then outcome measures should be measures of impairment and so forth. As most rehabilitation is concerned with the improvement of social participation, outcome measures should reflect changes in this domain: for example, how well does someone who forgets appointments now remember appointments? There are studies that directly assess such changes. For example, a study evaluating the use of a paging system for reducing everyday memory and planning problems (Wilson, Emslie, Quirk, & Evans, 2001), measured success in achieving everyday targets before, during, and after the provision of a pager.

Because of the great heterogeneity of patients receiving rehabilitation and because of the variety of aims and methods required to achieve ultimate goals, the measurement of treatment effectiveness and final outcomes resulting from rehabilitation are difficult to evaluate (Hart, 2017). It is now recognized that good evaluation of rehabilitation involves more than randomized controlled trials (Tate & Perdices, 2017). One of the most promising evaluation methods is the implementation of single-case experimental designs, which allow us to answer the question "Is this patient's improvement due to what we are doing or would it have happened anyway?" An important paper to appear by Tate and her colleagues (2016) is the SCRIBE statement (Single-Case Reporting guideline In Behavioural interventions), which provides standards for carrying out, reporting, and reviewing single-case experimental designs. This is surely one of the ways forward in evaluating the effectiveness of NR.

Case Study 3.1. Jose David: From Medical Student to Medical Anthropologist

We describe a case here to illustrate the process of rehabilitation for one of our patients, Jose David, a young man from Colombia, South America, who sustained an anoxic brain injury (Wilson & Jaramillo,

2014). He was in the third year of medical school in Bogotá, Colombia, and had been an "A" student in both his first and second years at medical school. He had also been an equestrian competitor since the age of 12, having ridden horses since he was 4 years old. Jose described himself as a sociable and friendly person who enjoyed spending time with his friends. As a result of an earlier horse-riding accident, he had a knee problem requiring surgery. Soon after the surgery, during the recovery period, he went into cardiac arrest. This was noticed by the staff, who began the recovery protocol immediately, calling for experienced staff to do this. Electroshock therapy was administered to restart the autonomous heart contractions. Records show that cardiac contractions stopped for around 2 minutes.

Jose David was taken to the intensive care unit where he stayed for 13 days. While there, he developed pneumonia. He then went to a general ward where he spent two more weeks before leaving the hospital. During this time, not only was he cared for by the hospital staff but his parents and friends also visited regularly to check on his progress. Jose David felt fine or else was denying any problems and thought he could return to his studies. He left the hospital to have Christmas at home with his family and began to study for his final exams that, due to the accident, had been postponed until the month after Christmas.

It was at this point that Jose David began to realize that he had difficulty remembering things and found it hard to study again. When he read something and tried to recall it, he found he could remember very little. As a consequence of this failure of his memory and attention, he believed he began to change as a person. He returned to the university and realized he could barely remember anything he had learned in the previous two years. He recalls, "It was shocking to get in front of a patient to practice a medical exam and not be able to do it correctly because I just didn't remember how it was done" (Wilson & Jaramillo, 2014, p. 64).

Jose had to withdraw from medical school and began a program designed for him by a team of health professionals in Bogotá. Another Colombian neuropsychologist, Dr. Patricia Montañes then saw Jose

David. She administered some tests and concluded that although there had been some improvement, there was still a deficiency in attention, concentration, and memory. She mentioned the Oliver Zangwill Centre (OZC) in England and so began the referral to our center in the United Kingdom.

Jose David himself described a conversation with his father that helped him realize he needed help, saying:

> "I have to mention the attitude that my family assumed toward my learning problem. I recall a talk I had with my father who with his vast experience of industrial and business planning but null on recovery therapies, once said 'When an engine is broken, it has to be fixed, but in order to have it properly fixed, spare parts have to be changed. What happened to you is probably the same, and as we are unable to change a spare part within your brain, what you need is to acquire the learning mechanisms which can help you cope and surpass your failure, but you need discipline and practice.' Thanks to this, and many more conversations we had, I realized help was needed. At first this was hard to accept, as it entailed many consequences which differed from what I had planned for my life. I had to withdraw from medical school and began a recovery program designed by a team of health professionals in Bogotá. It was composed of a phonoaudiologist [a speech and language therapist], an occupational therapist and a psychiatrist, all under the guidance of a neuropsychologist named Eugenia Solano. This recovery program lasted five months. During this time in the morning I did exercise, such as jogging and swimming on a daily basis. In the afternoon I attended therapy. These therapies were useful as they raised my self-esteem and security within myself." (in Wilson & Jaramillo, 2014, pp. 64–65)

We prefer not to see people from overseas as the second part of our program, the integration phase, means people come to the center for 2 days each week and the rest of the time they are integrating into work or education or at least into their own environments. Jose David had no relatives in England. His nearest relative, an aunt, lived in Switzerland, so it was not ideal. But with some pressure from his family and the fact that Jose David's English was excellent, we decided to admit him.

Initially Jose David came for a 3-day assessment. He was picked up at the apartment where he was staying and taken to the center to participate in the community meeting. This is a morning meeting attended by all clients, staff, and visitors to the center. It is loosely based on the morning meeting held at the Center in Phoenix run by Prigatano (1999) where one of us (Wilson) spent a sabbatical in 1993. This sabbatical was the stimulus for initiating the OZC.

The OZC staff and the assessments carried out by Dr. Monta-ñes demonstrated that Jose David had difficulty with both verbal and visual memory and with remembering to do things (prospective memory). There was also evidence of difficulties with attention/concentration and with visuospatial reasoning. In particular, Jose David had problems with sustained and divided attention, together with immediate and delayed recall of verbal and nonverbal material, recognition memory, and prospective memory. He was able to apply strategies to learn new material but this was inconsistent and he needed further help with this issue. Other cognitive skills appeared to be intact: Jose David had good verbal reasoning skills and his working memory (i.e., immediate or very short-term) was within normal limits. His speech, communication, and social cognition skills were appropriate.

Following the assessment, the team felt they could help Jose David and he, in turn, felt he would benefit from being at the center. A 6-week program was designed with the emphasis on study techniques, dealing with memory problems, and providing psychological support. The plan was submitted to Jose David's parents. They studied it and requested a few changes that were made.

The goals set with Jose David, his parents, and the OZC staff were as follows:

1. Identify his difficulties and his strengths and how these impact his day-to-day life (this goal was achieved by the end of the program).
2. Identify the implications of goal number one on a possible return to university (this goal was also achieved).
3. In a 40-minute period of studying technical material,

experience two or less attention slips (this goal was not achieved).

4. Demonstrate effective use of strategies for remembering textual information and demonstrate the use of these strategies on short stories and technical material (this goal was achieved).

5. Identify factors that contribute to his low mood (this goal was achieved).

6. Identify ways of coping with his low mood (this goal was achieved).

7. Use an external memory aid effectively at home and at the center (this goal was partially achieved).

For further details on these goals, see Wilson and Jaramillo (2014).

One of the study techniques taught (goal number four) and which has been used ever since is the PQRST (**P**review, **Q**uestion, **R**ead, **S**tate, and **T**est) strategy. This strategy, first described by Robinson (1970) was implemented through the use of flash cards, keeping an updated diary and setting goals. Studies evaluating the method are reported in Wilson (2009). The team, together with Jose David, recognized that he would not be able to study medicine again; as he showed an interest in economics, an application was made to study this at The School of African and Oriental Studies, which is part of London University. He was accepted and went there for 1 year during which time he kept in contact with the OZC mostly through regular e-mails, although he also visited us twice. Each of these 1-day reunions involved meetings with his therapists who learned of his progress and how he implemented the methods learned at the center.

After successfully obtaining a degree in economics, Jose David returned to Colombia and took first a bachelor's and then a master's degree in medical anthropology. He is hoping to complete a PhD soon. He still uses the PQRST without the T strategy for tasks that need to be accomplished within his professional career. He feels planning is important and uses the strategy daily without noticing; he feels it has become part of him. He is currently working as a lecturer at a university in Bogotá, and has carried out several important pieces of research on health issues such as teenage pregnancy myths and corruption within the public health of Colombia, for the controller´s office of Colombia. "For my dissertation in my undergraduate degree in anthropology, I conducted research on traditional healing remedies for malaria in the Pacific coast, and the dissertation for the master's degree was on narratives of HIV patients in Bogotá." Finally, Jose David is now married and has a daughter. Rehabilitation was both clinically and cost-effective in this case.

To comment further on this latter point, it is important that rehabilitation is cost-effective as well as clinically effective. Most countries are interested in whether or not rehabilitation is worth the effort in economic as well as clinical terms. Opinion is, perhaps, divided, with neurologists, neurosurgeons, and others more skeptical, while staff providing rehabilitation are more enthusiastic. Barnes (2016) said that clinical evidence supports rehabilitation and that short-term costs are offset by longer-term benefits. Furthermore, overall care costs have been shown to decrease after inpatient multidisciplinary team rehabilitation programs. Thus, optimal recovery results in significant savings in health care and social care costs. Some interesting work by Trexler and his colleagues in the United States (Trexler et al., 2010; Trexler, Parrott, & Malec, 2017) show that more people are likely to return to work after rehabilitation. For a recent review of evidence, see Worthington, da Silva Ramos, and Oddy (2017). We conclude this chapter with a quote from Wilson et al (2014):

> If the political will were there, and politicians could see the economic benefits to be gained from rehabilitation therapy, such treatment could be provided on a scale that would ensure that all who needed it could benefit to varying degrees, wherever they lived and whatever their financial circumstances. Personal, familial, communal and economic goals must be targeted in order to bring down costs and free people with brain injuries, as far as possible, from some of their disabling and burdensome problems that ultimately affect the well being of society as a whole. (p. 224).

CHAPTER 4

The Broad Theoretical Base of Neuropsychological Rehabilitation

Introduction

People with brain injury are likely to have several cognitive problems, particularly with attention, executive functions, memory, word finding, thinking, and reasoning. They are also likely to have emotional and behavioral problems such as anxiety, depression, social skills deficits, and so forth. Consequently, it is unlikely that any one theory, model, or framework can address all of these difficulties. Rehabilitation needs a broad theoretical base or several theoretical bases (Wilson, 2002). Hart et al. (2014) noted that rehabilitation is often said to be lacking in theories but, in fact, there are many theories that have influenced and continue to influence rehabilitation, as will be shown here.

What Are Theories and Models?

It is worth stating at this point what we understand by the terms "theory" and "model." The *Concise Oxford English Dictionary of Current English* (Allen, Fowler, & Fowler; 1990) says that a theory is "a supposition or system of ideas explaining something, especially one based on general principles independent of the particular thing to be explained" (p. 1,266). So, by "theory" we are referring to systems of ideas that are used to explain things such as why certain behaviors occur. A model is a representation to help us understand and predict related phenomena. Models range from simple analogies like explaining poor attention as being like a faulty switch, through to sophisticated and complex computer models used to explain how systems learn new information (Baddeley, 1993). Models and theories are often closely linked; for example, the Baddeley and Hitch working memory model (Baddeley & Hitch, 1974) also represents a theory of memory suggesting that there are three types of memory depending on the length of time or type of information that is stored.

Some Influential Theoretical Frameworks

Some of the most influential models and theories in NR over the past two decades are those of cognition, emotion, behavior, and learning. Several models of cognitive functioning have proved useful in rehabilitation, including models of language, reading, memory, attention, and perception. In addition, systemic models of intervention and team working have also been essential to the creation of NR.

Cognitive Neuropsychology

The most influential theories would appear to be those from cognitive neuropsychology, particularly from the fields of language and reading (see, e.g., Coltheart, Bates, & Castles, 1994; Mitchum & Berndt, 1995). Although it is true that theoretical models from cognitive neuropsychology have been highly influential in helping us understand and explain related phenomena and develop assessment procedures (Wilson & Patterson, 1990), Robertson (1991) argued that they offer little to our understanding of how to rehabilitate impaired functions. Wilson (1997) elaborates this point by explaining that because models from cognitive neuropsychology tell us *what* to treat and not *how* to treat, they are insufficient on their own to guide us through the many intricate processes involved in the rehabilitation process.

The Holistic Approach

Influenced by the work of Goldstein (1919, 1942), mentioned in Chapter 1, Diller (1976), Ben-Yishay (1978), and Prigatano (1986) pioneered the holistic approach, which is now seen as one of the most effective ways of providing cognitive rehabilitation to survivors of brain injury. This approach is currently much in evidence (Wilson et al., 2009). Holistic programs are concerned with increasing a client's awareness, alleviating cognitive deficits, developing compensatory skills, and providing vocational counselling. All such programs provide a mixture of individual and group therapy. They differ from the combined approach primarily in their recognition of the importance of treating emotional problems at the same time as treating cognitive and social difficulties.

Inherent in the holistic approach are theories and models of emotion, which are becoming increasingly important in cognitive rehabilitation, as evidenced, for example, by a special issue of the journal *Neuropsychological Rehabilitation* focusing entirely on biopsychosocial approaches in neuropsychological rehabilitation (Williams & Evans, 2003). Prigatano (1999) believes that dealing with the emotional effects of brain injury is essential to rehabilitation success. Social isolation, anxiety, and depression are common in survivors of an insult to the brain (Wilson, 2002). Gainotti (1993) distinguishes three main factors causing emotional and psychosocial problems after brain injury: those due to neurological factors, those due to psychological or psychodynamic factors, and those due to psychosocial factors. An example of the first might be someone with frontal lobe damage leading to loss of control and anger outbursts. An example of the second would be someone with reduced cognitive abilities and consequent loss of self-esteem together with depression because of an inability to engage in his or her previous profession. An example of the third might be someone who loses all his or her friends and colleagues following a brain injury and is thus very socially isolated. It is possible that these different types of emotional problems may overlap with each other. Other models and theories that need to be taken into account are those pertaining to premorbid personality; neurological, physical, and biochemical models; and models of emotional behavior such as those from cognitive-behavioral therapy (CBT).

A Recent Historical Viewpoint

Although the holistic approach (discussed above), advocated by Ben-Yishay (1978) and Prigatano (1986), is probably the preferred approach to NR at the present time, there is, of course, a history of theoretical influences in NR. In rehabilitation, models are useful for facilitating thinking about treatment, explaining treatment to therapists and relatives, and enabling us to conceptualize outcomes. NR comes from a diverse ancestry. Gianutsos (1991) suggests that cognitive rehabilitation is born of a mixed parentage, including neuropsychology, occupational therapy, speech and language therapy, and special education. Others refer to different fields: McMillan and Greenwood (1993), for example, believe that rehabilitation draws on clinical neuropsychology, behavioral analysis, cognitive retraining, and group and individual psychotherapy. Still others believe only one "parent'" is necessary, and these tend to be supporters of the use of theories from cognitive neuropsychology to inform treatment. Coltheart (1984), in the first issue of the journal *Cognitive Neuropsychology*, argues that rehabilitation programs should be based upon a theoretical analysis of the nature of the disorder to be treated. Mitchum and Berndt (1995) suggest that the goal of cognitive rehabilitation is "the development of rational therapies that are based upon a theoretical analysis of the nature of the disorder that is targeted for treatment" (p. 13). It is argued below that such theoretical analyses of cognitive functioning on their own are not sufficient to devise NR programs.

Theories and models from learning theory and behavioral psychology have also been used in rehabilitation since the 1970s (Ince, 1976; Lincoln, 1978), and in cognitive rehabilitation (Wilson, 1991). For example, behavioral assessments are employed in many cognitive programs to (1) identify and measure variables that control behavior, (2) select treatment, and (3) evaluate treatment. Numerous approaches from behavior therapy and behavior modification can and have been adopted for helping people with memory, perceptual, reading, and language disorders (Wilson, 1999). A behavioral analysis approach is usually incorporated into cognitive rehabilitation because it provides a structure, a way of analyzing cognitive problems, a means of assessing everyday manifestations of cognitive problems, and a means of evaluating the efficacy of treatment programs. It also, of course, supplies us with many existing treatment strategies such as shaping, chaining, modeling, desensitization, flooding, extinction, positive reinforcement, response cost, and so forth, all of which can be modified or adapted to suit particular rehabilitation purposes. Another attempt to develop a theory of NR is that of Gross and Schutz (1986). They propose five models of neuropsychological interventions, which can be helpful to clinicians in planning and delivering interventions:

1. The environmental control model
2. The stimulus–response (S-R) conditioning model
3. The skill training model
4. The strategy substitution model
5. The cognitive cycle model

Gross and Schutz claim that these models are hierarchical so that patients who cannot learn are treated with environmental control techniques; patients who can learn but cannot generalize need S-R conditioning; patients who can learn and generalize but cannot self-monitor should be given skill training; those who can self-monitor will benefit from strategy substitution; and those who can manage all of the above and are able to set their own goals will be best suited for treatment that is incorporated within the cognitive cycle model.

Although such a hierarchical model has a neatness about it, it is highly unlikely that absolute agreement would be found between therapists who were asked to make decisions about whether a particular patient could learn or generalize. Inability to learn cannot always be recognized with ease. We know that even comatose patients who have sustained a TBI are capable of some degree of learning (Boyle & Greer, 1983; Shiel et al., 1993). Furthermore, it is possible to teach generalization in many instances (Zarkowska, 1987). Despite these reservations, it can be argued that Gross and Schutz's models are useful in encouraging therapists to think about ways of tackling problems in rehabilitation.

In 1991 Coltheart stated that in order to treat a deficit, it is necessary to fully understand its nature, and to do this one has to have in mind how the function is normally achieved; and without this model one cannot determine what kinds of treatment would be appropriate. It is suggested that this approach is limited because, as stated earlier, people undergoing rehabilitation rarely have isolated deficits such as difficulty with reversible sentences; they may have emotional, social, and behavioral problems together with additional cognitive deficits; they are more likely to require help with the everyday problems caused by the deficit rather than help with the impairment, and understanding the deficit in detail (knowing *what* to do or treat) does not provide information on *how* to treat (see, e.g., Caramazza, 1989). We can conclude from this that theories of cognitive functioning are necessary but not sufficient in cognitive rehabilitation. Until we come up with a grand theory of rehabilitation encompassing cognition, emotion, behavior, new learning, recovery, and all the other factors of importance, no *one* theory is likely to be sufficient.

In 1993 Caramazza and Hillis wrote a paper entitled "For a Theory of Remediation of Cognitive Deficits." They pointed out that they were not concerned with the question of whether cognitive models are helpful in rehabilitation for "surely they are, [but] it is hard to imagine that efforts at therapeutic intervention would not be facilitated by having the clearest possible idea of what needs to be rehabilitated" (p. 218). Instead, they were concerned with the potential role of these models in articulating theoretically informed constraints on cognitive disorders. The belief that detailed assessment informed by theoretical cognitive models can identify "what needs to be rehabilitated" highlights, perhaps, the major difference between academic neuropsychologists engaged in cognitive rehabilitation and clinical neuropsychologists working at the "coal face." For those engaged in the day-to-day practice of helping people with cognitive deficits return to their most appropriate environments, relationships, and activities (arguably the main purpose of rehabilitation), "what needs to be rehabilitated" is *not* an impairment identified by a theoretically informed model but a real-life problem identified by the patient and his or her family. Such problems may well be caused by cognitive deficits but in most cases we do not try to rehabilitate the deficit so much as ease or overcome the everyday problems seen as important by the patient and his or her family (Wilson, 2002).

Do We Need Theoretical Models?

Does this mean theoretical models are not important? Of course not. Models of cognitive functioning have proved enormously helpful in identifying cognitive strengths and weaknesses, in explaining phenomena, and in making predictions about behavior. All are important features in designing and evaluating rehabilitation programs. They are not, however, sufficient on their own for designing NR programs. In reality a good NR program will draw on all of the models described above and apply them in an individual manner according to the client's presenting problems.

Theories and Models
for Teaching Compensatory Strategies

The earliest methods of cognitive rehabilitation drew on theories of learning and behavior therapy. For example, one of the most commonly used rehearsal strategies in cognitive rehabilitation, the PQRST method, first described by Robinson (1970), comes from the field of study techniques. Similarly, the work of Glisky, Schacter, and Tulving (1986), using the method of vanishing cues to train computer skills, and the evidence base regarding the use of expanded rehearsal/ spaced retrieval and verbal mnemonics all have a theoretical basis in behavioral techniques (Wilson, 2009).

Perhaps one of the most influential models used to aid cognitive rehabilitation in everyday clinical practice is the approach for training compensatory aids by Sohlberg and colleagues (1994). The authors find that the "Sohlberg approach" is regularly referenced by clinicians as the model they use to implement cognitive rehabilitation. The approach advocates a three-phase training model:

1. The first phase is an awareness training phase, in which patients' insight into their cognitive deficits is raised and they learn the purpose and function of compensatory aid systems.
2. The second phase is the practice training phase, where the patient practices implementing his or her compensatory aid system in simulated situations.
3. The third is the generalization phase, where patients learn to use their compensatory system in novel contexts and real-life situations.

Sohlberg and colleagues (1994) explain that "although presented as a linear three-stage rehabilitation model, in practice the different stages of training may be cycled through several times or even implemented concurrently depending on the needs and progress of the individual patient" (p. 17). Even though the three-phase model was originally conceived for compensatory memory aids, and therefore is underpinned by theories of memory impairment and learning theory, it is now widely recognized in clinical practice as a generic model for training compensatory aids for any type of cognitive deficit (e.g., executive, attention, memory, or visual–spatial compensatory aids). It is noteworthy that implicit within the model is the notion that psychological and emotional factors mediate successful utilization of compensatory aids and that a holistic approach to training should be adhered to, although this is not referenced in the theoretical background postulated in the text (see Sohlberg et al., 1994).

Theories and Models of Emotion

The management and remediation of the emotional consequences of brain injury have become increasingly important over the past 20 years. Prigatano (1999) suggests that rehabilitation is likely to fail if we do not deal with emotional issues. Bowen et al. (1998) found that 38% of survivors of TBI experienced mood disorders. Judd and Wilson (2005) surveyed practitioners in the United Kingdom to find the main challenges faced when establishing a therapeutic alliance with brain-injured patients requiring help with emotional difficulties. Cognitive, behavioral, and emotional reasons were the most likely to affect therapeutic alliances.

Ever since Beck's highly influential book *Cognitive Therapy and the Emotional Disorders* appeared in 1976, CBT has become one of the most important and best-validated psychotherapeutic procedures. An update of Beck's model appeared in 1996 (Salkovskis, 1996). CBT has been one of the key underlying models used to address emotional needs in NR since its inception, and was rated the number one model used in clinical neuropsychology by a national survey of practitioners in the United Kingdom (Wilson et al., 2008). There is discrepant evidence regarding the effectiveness of CBT when used to treat people with ABI. For instance, Lincoln and Flannaghan (2003) found that CBT for stroke survivors was not effective. However, closer analysis of the treatment protocol reveals that the lack of effect is more likely to be a feature of the length of treatment and quality of the intervention (i.e., highly protocolized intervention, not tailored to the clients' individual needs). In contrast, Fann, Hart, and Schomer (2009) found in their systematic review of evidence since the 1980s that CBT for depression following TBI appeared to have better results than pharmacological interventions.

In clinical practice, most clinicians recognize that CBT requires adaptation for neurological populations and the intervention should be conducted in the context of a wider holistic interdisciplinary intervention (Ownsworth & Gracey, 2017). However, there have been limited publications about its adapted use with neurological populations until relatively recently. Williams, Evans, and Wilson (2003) illustrate the use of CBT with survivors of TBI, and Tyerman and King (2004) provide a good account of its use in the context of treating adjustment disorders following ABI.

The diagnostic construct of an adjustment disorder as a model of explaining emotional disturbance following ABI is widely utilized in clinical practice, as illustrated in Tyerman and King's chapter on the topic (2004). However, it is noteworthy that in our clinical experience, brain injury survivors often suffer from chronic adjustment disorders (i.e., symptoms last more than 3 months after the brain injury). Adjustment difficulties are also one of the primary barriers to change in rehabilitation, yet chronic adjustment disorder is not a recognized condition in DSM-5 or ICD-11. In fact, according to these diagnostic manuals, if the symptoms last longer than 6 months the diagnostic category "adjustment disorder" should not be used at all. The assumption is that people with symptoms lasting more than 6 months would be more likely to meet criteria for depression (Patra & Sarkar, 2013). This is not our clinical experience for the neurological population. Often these clients do not meet criteria for depression or anxiety, or any other psychiatric diagnosis. The removal of "chronic" as a subtype of adjustment disorder in the new diagnostic manuals means that these clients can struggle to access services because entry into psychological services is often based on formal psychiatric diagnosis. This leads to clients being inappropriately diagnosed as depressed in order to access services. The authors agree with Kazlauskas and colleagues (2018), who argue that more empirical evidence from clinical practice is required to help develop the model of adjustment disorder.

One influential model from recent years that addresses the issue of adjustment in neurological populations, is the Y-shaped model (Gracey et al., 2009). This model suggests that "a complex and dynamic set of biological, psychological and social factors interact to determine the consequences of acquired brain injury" (p. 867). The model integrates findings from psychosocial adjustment, awareness, and well-being. It is, essentially, an attempt to reduce the discrepancy between the old "me" and the current "me" into the "new" me. One of the important aspects of the Y-shaped model is that it describes consolidation of new, adaptive, and positive meanings in life, highlighting the importance of ending therapy with a sense of starting a journey, rather than having completed one (Ownsworth & Gracey,

2017). Addressing issues in identity has become increasingly important in rehabilitation. Ownsworth (2014) covers this work in depth in
her excellent book *Self-Identity after Brain Injury*, and mentions some
important theories of identity including those of Tajfel and Turner
(1979) and Jetten, Haslam, and Haslam (2012).

Analytic psychotherapy is also used in NR practice, and Prigatano
(1999) is one of the best-known original advocates of this approach
with survivors of brain injury. More recently the use of this approach
has been developed via the theoretical framework known as neuro-
psychoanalysis (Kaplan-Solms, 2018); and there is a growing body of
evidence to support its utility in NR (Schönberger, Yeates, & Hobbs
(in press)). For useful resources related to this theoretical framework,
see *www.neuro-psa.org.uk*).

Other Theories and Models

Other attempts to tackle theoretical specification of rehabilitation
processes include Sohlberg and Mateer (2001), Tate, Taylor, and Aird
(2013), and Hart (2009). The Tate et al. paper describes the Model for
Assessing Treatment Effectiveness (MATE), which was designed to
bridge the gap between research methodologies and clinical practice.
It incorporates the ICF classification of functioning, disability, and
health together with elements of single-case experimental designs. It
is a seven-level hierarchical framework, ranging from level 0, denot-
ing no treatment, through intermediate levels that might include a
generic assessment pre- and postapplication of an uncontrolled treatment (level 4). The highest level is 6, a program involving assessment
using both generic and targeted measures prior to and after the introduction of a controlled procedure. The MATE gives helpful directions
toward how treatment may be improved.

An interesting approach from the Moss Rehabilitation Research
Institute (Hart et al., 2014) attempts to provide a taxonomy of rehabilitation treatments. They are concerned with theories of treatment
and want to structure some order from the chaos of the multitude of

rehabilitation interventions. This is explained in Hart (2017). Their taxonomy is a "framework by which rehabilitation treatments may be characterized using *treatment theory*, a concept introduced in the context of rehabilitation by Keith and Lipsey (1993)." They suggest that all interventions may be characterized by specifying three things: the target, the active ingredients, and the mechanism of actions, all of which are measurable.

Clinical Practice in the United Kingdom

Because survivors of brain injury are likely to have both a mixture of cognitive and noncognitive problems, no one theory, model, or framework is sufficient to deal with the range, or indeed complexity, of problems faced by those requiring cognitive rehabilitation. In Diller's words, "While current accounts of remediation have been criticised as lacking a theoretical base, it might be more accurate to state that remediation must take into account several theoretical bases" (Diller, 1987, p. 9). We need to have some understanding of theories of assessment, recovery, learning, personality, and plasticity to name but a few. In an attempt to illustrate the complexity of rehabilitation and to persuade those who think one theoretical approach is sufficient, Wilson (2002) published a provisional model of cognitive rehabilitation in which she synthesized a number of existing models and approaches.

Wilson et al. (2008) wanted to find out how Wilson's (2002) model applied to practicing British psychologists working in brain injury rehabilitation. They devised a questionnaire based on the model. Assessment, treatment, and evaluation practices were surveyed together with theories and models influencing clinical practice. Fifty-four clinical neuropsychologists took part. Responses to 20 questions were calculated, providing descriptive statistics. All participants reported assessing the cognitive, emotional, and psychosocial consequences of brain injury. Fifty-seven different models and theories in eight categories were cited by clinicians as influencing their clinical practice. CBT was alluded to most frequently. Most clinicians had access to information on gross structural brain damage from CT scans; few had access to other imaging techniques such as fMRI. The conclusions were that clinical neuropsychologists in the United Kingdom referred to a range of theoretical approaches in their work; CBT was the most popular, and all parts of Wilson's synthesized model were used by some people. At least three questions arose from this study: first, what were the models and theories cited; second, why were there so many different models used; and third, why was CBT the most popular model?

Which Models and Theories Were Used in Clinical Practice?

The authors recognized that their survey was not necessarily a completely accurate reflection of the participants' clinical practice but rather a summary of how they *perceived* their practice. It is also possible that some respondents might have said what they thought the interviewer wanted to hear although attempts were made to avoid leading questions by providing yes/no choices (or several choices) to the factual questions. In addition, many participants were self-critical, so it was believed that the answers were not simply given to please the interviewer.

Not all respondents were clear about the differences between a model, a theory, and therapeutic practice. Indeed, several people reported therapeutic strategies in reply to the question about which models most influenced their clinical practice even though these are not, strictly speaking, models or theories. We included them in the analysis, however, as it may be that a future study will want to consider these approaches when looking at the practice of clinical neuropsychology. Nevertheless, 57 different models and theories were identified and these were grouped into eight categories following perusal of the literature and discussion with colleagues. In order of the frequency in which these were endorsed, theories and models of emotion and therapy came top with over 35% of people saying that they used these in clinical practice. This category included CBT and psychodynamic approaches. Second in frequency came models and theories of neuropsychology and cognition with 26% endorsing these. Working memory and the supervisory attention system were cited here. Almost 18% of the participants endorsed models and theories of behavior and learning with such examples as learning theory or errorless learning. Over 9% mentioned holistic and other broad-based treatments such as Prigatano's principles and Wilson's model. Nearly 4% cited health, general adjustment, and coping, giving as examples rational optimism and interpersonal approaches. The same number mentioned "others"; this included risk assessment and insight. Just over 3% declared anatomy and neuroplasticity, using these two terms. Finally, less than 1% stated development with the terms "lifespan development" or "child development."

To conclude, in the words of Alan Baddeley (personal communication), "A good theory teaches us to doubt." We need to know when we are wrong and we need to challenge theories in order to improve science. A model allows us to test out the various components, find double dissociations, and prove whether our hypotheses are true or not. In NR we need to draw on a number of theories, models, and frameworks or else we risk bad clinical practice.

CHAPTER 5

Appropriate Assessment and Formulation for Neuropsychological Rehabilitation

Introduction

In this chapter we consider the meaning of assessment, the purposes of assessment, different approaches to assessment, a comparison between standardized and functional assessments, and why assessments are needed to plan rehabilitation. We shall review assessments of cognitive functioning, emotion and mood, psychosocial functioning, and challenging behaviors. Results of different kinds of assessment can be assembled to provide a detailed, single, and coherent formulation that can supply a framework for individualized interventions. Visually presenting assessment results in this manner helps summarize information, which in turn helps promote a shared understanding among a team of clinicians. It is argued that equipped with such understanding, clinicians can offer more effective and appropriate interventions.

The Meaning and Purposes of Assessment

Assessment is concerned with judgment, estimation, appraisal, analysis, and evaluation (Wilson, 2009). Psychological assessment has been described as a testing procedure using a combination of techniques to help produce certain hypotheses about a person and his or her behavior, personality, and capabilities (Framingham, 2016). This definition, however, is perhaps rather less comprehensive than an older, but possibly more apt, definition by Sundberg and Tyler (1962) when they pointed out that assessment involves the systematic collection, organization, and interpretation of information about a person and his or her situation.

Obviously, the manner in which the above process is conducted will depend upon the main purpose of the assessment. In rehabilitation, we may want to assess a patient in order to provide a map of a person's strengths and weaknesses, or to predict future behaviors or to answer certain questions such as "What is this person's level of cognitive functioning and has it declined from the premorbid level?" We may want to know if a failure on a visual perceptual test is due to poor acuity or to an actual perceptual disorder. If we identify memory problems, we need to know if the memory difficulty is restricted to a certain modality or if it is global. We may want to know if a problem behavior is more likely to occur when a particular member of staff is on duty or if it changes when the person is hungry or tired. Bigler (2012) said that neuropsychological assessment measures cognitive and neurobehavioral functioning in order to make neuropsychological inferences and diagnostic conclusions. In practice, particularly when one is concerned with rehabilitation, there are many other reasons for carrying out an assessment. Malec (2017) noted that "rehabilitation is best planned based on a very comprehensive, holistic assessment of the person's strengths and limitations as well as the social and physical environment in which they live" (p. 36). It can be seen then that different measurement tools are required depending on the overriding reason for the assessment. We now consider three types of assessment procedures: (1) standardized tests; (2) behavioral assessments/observations; and (3) self-report measures. Then we examine the method used to formulate this information into a coherent and holistic hypothesis drawing on neuropsychological theory and principles. The resulting formulation is used to guide the neuropsychological rehabilitation plan.

Standardized Tests

Standardized neuropsychological tests include psychometric models based on statistical analyses; localization methods that attempt to determine which part of the brain is damaged; assessments derived from theoretical models of cognitive functioning; exclusion model— that is to say, assessments that exclude certain reasons for the problem (e.g., excluding poor eyesight and naming problems when diagnosing visual object agnosia); and ecological models, which predict problems in real life (Wilson, 1996b).

A standardized test must always be administered and scored in exactly the same way. It allows one to compare the score obtained to a criterion. The person or people devising the test will have set a procedure for administration; they will have developed a scoring method and collected norms. They will also have collected evidence of the consistency, that is to say, the reliability of the test as well as its usefulness. They will have addressed validity—that is, they will have demonstrated that the test actually measures what it purports to measure, and they will have prepared a detailed manual. The test user needs to know what the test is for and how good a measure it is; whether it is suitable for the patients one is planning to assess; how to administer and score the test; and how to make sense of the results.

Certain questions can be answered through the use of standardized tests; others need functional or behavioral assessments (to be discussed later). Until the late 1970s the main questions neuropsychologists were expected to answer were those that supported decisions made by neurologists and neurosurgeons. Examples might be "Which part of the brain has been affected?"; "Are language functions located in the left hemisphere as we would expect or is there a different representation?"; "Are there any cognitive deficits?"

Recently, and partly because of neuroimaging techniques, the earlier questions are not sufficient. Today we have more models of neuropsychological assessment and therefore more reasons for measuring areas such as cognitive functioning, emotions, behavior, and psychosocial functioning. The types of questions that can now be answered by standardized tests include:

1. What is this person's general level of intellectual functioning?
2. What was the probable level of premorbid functioning?
3. What are this person's cognitive strengths and weaknesses?
4. How does this person's memory/language/perceptual/executive functioning compare with people of the same age in the general population?
5. Is the level of functioning consistent with what one would expect from the person's level of intellectual ability?
6. Is the memory problem global or restricted to certain kinds of material (e.g., is memory for visual material better than for verbal material)?
7. Does this person have a high level of anxiety?
8. Is this person depressed?

These are the kinds of questions clinical neuropsychologists typically address when carrying out a neuropsychological assessment and they can, to a large extent, be answered through the administration of standardized tests provided they have been adequately normed and have been shown to be reliable and valid. Answering such questions requires the information gathered to be evaluated using a process of neuropsychological formulation (see section on neuropsychological formulation below).

There are, however, other important rehabilitation questions that standardized tests cannot answer or can only answer indirectly. These include questions such as:

1. What problems do the patient and family find most distressing?
2. How do the identified cognitive problems manifest themselves in everyday life?
3. Is this person safe to return home?
4. How should we teach the use of a compensatory aid?
5. What level of support is available at home?

6. Are the problems exacerbated by depression or anxiety?

7. What is this person's cultural background?

In order to answer these and similar questions one needs to use a different kind of approach.

Functional or Behavioral Assessments

Although standardized tests enable us to build up a map of a person's cognitive strengths and weaknesses, they are insufficient to help us plan rehabilitation. The standardized tests provide information that can stop us asking the cognitively impossible of a patient: thus we need to know, for example, whether or not the person concerned will be able to understand instructions, remember things, have problems reading, and so forth. But they will not tell us what problems are most distressing for the patients and their families, what coping methods are used, what is the best intervention strategy to adopt, and how to determine whether our treatment programs are effective? We need, therefore, to complement our standardized tests with other forms of assessment. We need to assess real-life functioning. To some extent, standardized ecologically valid tests such as the Rivermead Behavioural Memory Test-3 (Wilson et al., 2008) or the Test of Everyday Attention (Robertson, Ward, Ridgeway, & Nimmo-Smith, 1994) can do this, because an ecologically valid test assesses and predicts real-life or everyday problems. These tests, however, do not specify in sufficient detail the problems we need to identify in order to select or develop relevant treatment in rehabilitation. In order to do this, we need to measure behavior that occurs directly in daily life. As with standardized assessments, behavioral measures are concerned with the systematic collection, organization, and interpretation of details about a person and his or her situation.

The two means of assessment differ in their implementation. The core of a behavioral assessment is the analysis of a person's behavior, its antecedents, and its consequences. This is often described as an ABC assessment or a functional analysis. Thus, if someone is refusing to participate in a group session, we may want to know if this is trig-gered by fear of failure, social anxiety, fatigue, dislike of the other people present, lack of understanding, or some other factor. These are the antecedent factors. What behavior does the person exhibit? Is it shouting, swearing, withdrawing into themselves, or running out of the room? What are the consequences? Is the person removed from the group, allowed to sit next to a friend, or taught some anxiety man-agement techniques? These are some of the reasons why a functional or ABC analysis should be conducted. Behavioral assessment proce-dures have provided those of us in NR with a number of techniques for measuring behavior. Wilson (2009) outlines these in some detail. Here we focus on observations; self-report measures, including ques-tionnaires, rating scales, and diaries; and behavioral interviews with patients, family members, and staff.

Observations

Observations in the natural environment are important. Because the purpose of rehabilitation is to improve functioning in everyday life, we often need to observe patients in everyday life. Observations may reveal behavior that is not detected by assessments, interviews, ques-tionnaires, rating scales, or checklists. Through observation, one can also recognize events leading up to a problem and the consequences maintaining a behavior, as well as further assist in carrying out a func-tional analysis. Not all behaviors are amenable to observation because observation itself might lead to changes in behavior or because the behavior of concern is about attitudes, beliefs, or feelings. Rating scales, questionnaires, or self-report measures may need to be used here. These are discussed below. Sometimes it makes sense to design a simulated situation such as a mock office, shop, or kitchen for the pur-pose of observation. Such observations are worth considering when one wants to measure an infrequent behavior such as a low-frequency anger outburst or when one is short of time or can only observe in a restricted range of situations. It is always possible that simulated situ-ations may lead to inaccurate information, but if one is reasonably confident that the simulated and naturalistic situations are close, then they can be a very useful tool for eliciting a better understanding of what difficulties an individual may face in a real-life setting, but without the associated risks. For example, a nurse wanting to return to work after suffering an ABI might be provided with a simulated situation to practice taking people's blood pressure to evaluate whether any mistakes occur, as failure to do this correctly in a real-world setting could result in harm to a patient.

Observations may involve any one of the following, or combination of the following methodologies.

1. *Continuous recording*, whereby one measures everything the person does including all movements, words, activities, and so forth. In practice, this is often difficult or impossible to do although one could use video recording here so that one is able to play the tape many times over.

2. *Event recording*, whereby one notes each time the behavior of interest occurs, such as the number of times someone forgets to take medication or shouts during a therapy session. This may be hard to do for high-frequency behaviors but be perfectly possible for certain other behaviors such as stopping a particular task during a work placement. In practice, event recording is usually confined to certain periods of the day or week such as during an occupational therapy session or during lunch break. This recording method can also lead to inaccuracy if one is sampling a period when the behavior is more or less likely to occur.

3. *Duration recording*, which refers to situations when one wants to know how long a certain behavior lasts. For example, if we need to know how long it takes someone to get dressed or for how long someone is screaming, then duration recording might be the method of choice. One disadvantage is that it is not always easy to determine when a particular behavior starts and stops. For example, if one is measuring "time on task" and the person stops to look at the ceiling, it may not be clear whether the person is thinking about the next step or has lost concentration.

4. *Interval recording*, which is a convenient method of sampling

behavior. The total observation period is divided into time intervals and the observer notes whether or not the target behavior occurs at all during that time interval. This method is particularly useful for certain behaviors such as repetition of a story, question, or joke. A further advantage is that it can indicate both the severity and duration of a behavior. A major disadvantage, however, is that it is an *estimate* and not an accurate recording of the frequency of the target behavior. If repetition of a question occurs at all in the interval it will be noted, but the note does not distinguish between one or two repetitions and several repetitions. In practice, clinicians may combine interval recording and event recording, so that if one samples repetition behavior for a 15-minute interval four times a day, one could note *how many* (event recording) repetitions occur during that interval.

5. *Time sampling*, whereby the observer records at the end of a predetermined interval, say every hour *on* the hour. The length of the interval depends on the target behavior itself and the time available to the observer. Thus, one might decide to observe whether or not a person is calm at the end of every 15-minute period during the morning or whether the person is present for meals at the start of every meal. The advantage of this method is that it does not require continuous monitoring, although it does require precise timing in order to avoid biasing the results.

Self-Report Measures: Questionnaires, Rating Scales, and Checklists

Measures of this nature have been used since the early days of psychology (e.g., Galton, 1907). Questionnaires, rating scales, and checklists can be applied in *cognitive assessment* (Broadbent, Cooper, Fitzgerald, & Parks, 1982; Simblett, Ring, & Bateman, 2017); for *emotional problems* (Zigmond & Snaith, 1983); *behavior problems* (Kelly et al., 2017); *sexual problems* (Knight et al., 2008); and *psychosocial functioning* (Tate et al., 2012). The European Brain Injury Questionnaire (EBIQ; Teasdale et al., 1997) covers all of these areas and is a psychometrically robust instrument (Bateman, Teasdale, & Willmes, 2009; Tate, 2010). Tate (2010) provides an excellent summary of many of these measures together with a comment on their psychometric properties. Of course, patients with cognitive problems may not have good insight and may not therefore always be aware of the nature of their difficulties. They may not remember them, they may deny them, they may be unaware of them, or not recognize their importance. Nevertheless, we can determine how people *perceive* their problems and thereby obtain some idea of their level of insight. Family members, caretakers, and other professional staff involved may have a better understanding and we may well want to ask these significant others to complete rating scales, checklists, or questionnaires. Is there a discrepancy between the results of the patient and the significant other or not? If so, we can make an educated guess as to the reliability of the significant other. Olsson et al. (2006), found a good degree of consistency between self-ratings and significant other ratings among 30 people with brain injury and their caregivers on a modified version of the Everyday Memory Questionnaire (Sunderland, Harris, & Baddeley, 1983). Checklists can provide additional information to that obtained from questionnaires and rating scales.

Self-Monitoring Techniques

While these are yet another of the self-report measures, they differ because they require continuous monitoring rather than completion of a prepared questionnaire, checklist, or rating scale. Because of this difference we are considering self-monitoring separately. As far back as 1970, Kanfer said that observing one's own behavior (self-monitoring) can lead to increases or decreases in that behavior. Recording the amount of alcohol one consumes, for example, can lead to a reduction in the amount that has been consumed. Self-monitoring is sometimes used in NR, typically to try to obtain a record of the problem being treated. Patients may be asked to complete a diary, recording each time they take medication, have a seizure, or get lost on a journey. Once again, the problem with using self-monitoring for people with brain injury is that they may forget to record incidents. Sometimes this omission can be overcome through training. Alderman, Fry, and Youngson (1995) describe how they taught a brain-injured patient to improve her self-monitoring; Kime, Lamb, and Wilson (1996) improved self-monitoring in an amnesic patient; and in our clinical practice, we have improved self-monitoring of anxiety and fatigue.

Behavioral Interviews

The purpose of a behavioral interview is to gain an understanding of the antecedents of the problem behavior, to describe the behavior precisely and unambiguously, and to identify the consequences that maintain the behavior. A chapter on the empowerment behavioral management approach (Betteridge, Cotterill, & Murphy, 2017) describes how this can be carried out in clinical practice with one woman who was smoking 60 cigarettes a day. Such interviews can be helpful in problem behaviors, enabling one to identify questions or situations that trigger and maintain a problem behavior. One example (see Wilson, 2009) was the patient CW, who was left with a very severe amnesia after herpes simplex viral encephalitis, and who felt constantly as if he had just woken up and frequently said that his situation was "like being dead." Typically, he would say, "This is the first taste I've had, the first sight I've had, it's like being dead." If people sympathized with him or repeated back to him "So it feels like being dead?," he became more and more agitated. Certain questions triggered this behavior, as did memory tests. These were the antecedents. The behavior was the statement "It's like being dead." The consequences maintaining the behavior were responses indicating sympathy or empathy. The problem was reduced when caregivers or therapists changed the subject so instead of sympathizing, asked him something he was comfortable with, such as "What age should a child start to learn to play music?" or "What is the best instrument for a child to learn to play?" Questions like this calmed him down and the same soothing questions could be asked as often as necessary, as CW did not remember he had been asked the same things earlier. Behavioral interviewing may not lead to accurate information, as people may forget what their problems are or, as we have said before, their insight may be poor. Here one may also wish to interview the relatives, caregivers, and therapists who may be aware of related situations and can give more accurate information.

A Comparison of Standardized
and Behavioral Assessments

In 1968, Mischel discussed the differences between these two types
of assessment. On the whole, standardized tests tend to tell us what a
person *has*. Thus, a person may *have* a visual object agnosia or unilateral neglect or a surface dyslexia. Behavioral assessments, on the other
hand, tend to tell us what a person *does*. Thus, a person with unilateral
neglect may bump into doorways, trap his or her hands in the wheelchair spokes, and leave food on the left-hand side of the plate.

Standardized tests typically see the observed behavior as a *sign,*
so if someone is unable to complete a cancellation test, omitting many
of the targets on the left-hand side, this is a sign of unilateral neglect,
whereas in a behavioral assessment the observed behavior is seen as a
sample, so we are sampling, for example, whether the person neglects
things on the left in real life.

Implicit in the traditional approach is the view that the results
from an assessment are a reflection of the underlying problem. Implicit
in the behavioral approach is the assumption that behavior is a result
of environmental circumstances. So, the former kind of assessment
assumes that the behavior observed is relatively stable; a person's IQ,
for example, will not fluctuate a great deal if measured in the morning
or in the evening. This is sometimes true for patients seen in rehabilitation. Thus, someone with the amnesic syndrome will be unable
to recall new material whenever tested, but someone with unilateral
neglect may vary depending on the presence of fatigue, anxiety, stress,
or where the material is positioned. These variables would be looked
at in a behavioral assessment.

Another difference is that a traditional assessment is carried out
only once, the more functional assessments are typically carried out
several times in different situations. In standardized tests, the relationship with treatment is *indirect;* as one does not, or should not, treat
someone in order for that person to pass a test. Behavioral approaches,
in contrast, have a much more *direct* relationship to treatment: for
example, if we are measuring how many times someone catches his

or her hand in the wheelchair spokes, we would almost certainly be treating this problem, and the measurement will continue in both the baseline and treatment period.

Finally, standardized assessments are typically performed *prior* to treatment. They may sometimes be conducted during or following treatment to help raise a person's insight or awareness of cognitive deficits in function. For example, patients may report they have made a "full recovery" and "don't need cognitive rehab" or claim their previous results are invalid because they "weren't trying." Repeat testing can be set up as a therapeutic task to help raise a patient's insight into his or her cognitive deficits. In the authors' experience, patients often consent to the reassessment, as they are motivated to see "whether anything has changed" or whether when giving their best effort their performance is better. The clinician often knows the patient's cognition is unlikely to have changed from the previous assessment but it is important for the patient's psychological well-being to reach this realization for him- or herself. Just telling a patient this information only serves to reinforce defensive denial of deficits.

Often patients have undergone testing prior to their admission to rehabilitation but it is not possible to simply use the previous assessment to aid this process of insight raising. This is because patients may not remember the assessment and therefore are skeptical about the validity of the results. If the results are discussed with patients while the emotional salience of the experience of failure is fresh in their mind, the authors find patients are more accepting of the findings. Discussion about how the person is performing compared to age-matched peers is a helpful way of helping the person understand their cognitive deficits. This, in turn, can help raise insight into their need for a compensatory aid. The use of standardized assessment, therapeutically in this way, is part of the Sohlberg approach to training people to use a compensatory aid, and interested readers should refer to this manual for useful aids to implement this intervention (Sohlberg et al., 1994). However, it should be noted that standardized assessments *are not usually part of the treatment process itself,* whereas behavioral assessments can be seen as an essential part of the treatment process.

Case Study 5.1. Assessment in a Life-or-Death Decision-Making Process

In the United Kingdom, it is possible for hospitals and families to apply to the courts for permission to remove food and water so as to let a person die if this person has been in a vegetative state for many months. People in a minimally conscious state and therefore with limited self-awareness are not allowed to die in this way. Shiel and Wilson were asked to see such a person, a young woman, in the late 1990s (Shiel & Wilson, 1998). In fact, this person had already been seen by McMillan (1996). The background was as follows: the young woman had been involved in a traffic accident at the age of 22 years and had sustained a very severe TBI. Apparently, she had told her family that if she were severely brain-damaged she would not want to live. A medical person had examined the young woman on one occasion only and concluded there was no evidence of cognition. McMillan then assessed her 26-months postinjury and found that the patient was sentient, was not vegetative and, at the time of testing, wanted to live. Thus, there was a difference of judgment between the medical assessor and the neuropsychologist. Shiel and Wilson were asked to give a second opinion. On seeing the young woman in the hospital, certain biographical facts were obtained and individual members of the staff working closely with the patient were asked if they had a way of communicating with her. The following means of communication were described by the nurse and the occupational therapist:

1. Eye contact
2. Smile
3. Frown
4. Long blink for "yes"
5. Thumbs up for "yes" and down for "no"
6. Pointing when given a choice of two items
7. Waving goodbye
8. Pointing to where she felt pain
9. Attempting to push away (nurse only)
10. Nodding and shaking head (nurse only)

11. Raising eyebrows for "no" (nurse only)
12. Shrugging shoulders (nurse only)
13. Withdrawal by closing her eyes (occupational therapist only)
14. Bemused expression (occupational therapist only)
15. Using a switch (occupational therapist only)

Shiel and Wilson (1998) assessed the woman 12 times over 2 days in carefully balanced trials. She clearly indicated that she wanted to live. The case was dropped and the patient allowed to live. She was followed up by McMillan and Herbert 5 and 10 years later (McMillan & Herbert, 2004). Although she remained very impaired, she could hold a simple conversation and showed evidence of continuing recovery. What was worrying initially was that an eminent medical doctor had determined there was no evidence of cognition; he only saw her on one occasion and this may well have been when she was sleepy and unresponsive.

The work involved in this case was partly responsible for changes in assessment. Patients with a disorder of consciousness are now assessed over a prolonged period of observation, typically 6 weeks by at least two independent doctors and their findings should be supported by the observations of all professionals and family members in contact with the patient (Bates, 2005). Observations should take place at different times of the day, when the patient is in different positions, and the observations of everybody in contact with the patient should be recorded and taken into account.

Neuropsychological Formulation

Formulation refers to the process of applying theory and empirical knowledge to information gathered via assessment to derive hypotheses concerning the nature, causes, and factors influencing a patient's current problems or behavioral presentation/situation. During the process of formulation the multitude of possible influences on an individual's level of functioning and psychological state are considered. The hypotheses generated are used to guide further assessment and/

or inform the rehabilitation plan (see British Psychological Society, 2011).

Neuropsychological formulation is guided principally by the empirical and theoretical literature regarding cognitive functioning (e.g., cognitive models and neuroanatomical models of cognitive abilities such as memory, attention, and executive functions), and applies biopsychosocial and systemic models to aid understanding of an individual's behavioral presentation. There are two stages at which neuropsychological formulation should occur: first, during the analysis of standardized (i.e., psychometric) neuropsychological test results, especially when these are being used to help differentially diagnose a patient's presenting problems; and second, prior to the NP planning process. The approach commonly utilized in clinical practice to aid the formulation process at each of these stages is described below.

Formulation of Neuropsychological Assessment

Prior to commencing NR, formal standardized psychometric assessment is usually conducted to clarify diagnosis or to understand an individual's cognitive profile after an ABI. The objective is to determine the extent to which an individual's pattern of cognitive strengths and weaknesses are attributable to organic versus psychological or extraneous factors (e.g., culture, effort). This information is then used to inform the NR program. In this context, the process of neuropsychological assessment and formulation are intertwined. The neuropsychologist engages in a process of progressive hypothesis testing from beginning to end. For instance, an initial hypothesis is formed based on information gathered from the clinical interview and background information provided in the referral documentation. This informs the battery of psychometric tests that are selected for administration, although it is also generally considered good practice to ensure that each core cognitive domain is assessed (see Figure 5.1).

Figure 5.1 details the core cognitive domains that need to be considered during a neuropsychological assessment. The items in the outer dark gray borders represent domains that need to be held in

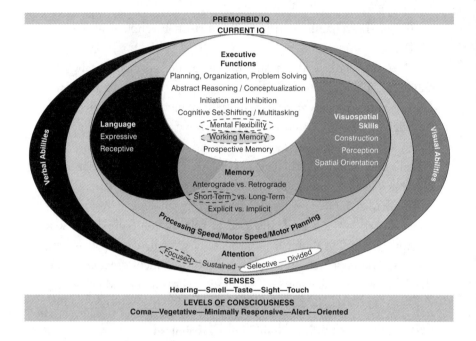

FIGURE 5.1. Core cognitive domains model.

mind throughout the assessment process. For example, when selecting or evaluating an assessment tool designed to assess a specific cognitive domain, it needs to be considered in the context of the impact these factors might have on the person's performance (e.g., the assessor should hold in mind the person's estimated premorbid IQ and any disorder of consciousness that might compromise the person's ability to engage in the assessment).

Fundamentally, this diagram illustrates that no cognitive ability exists in isolation, they are all interdependent on each other, with some domains (e.g., attention and processing speed) forming the foundations that higher-level skills (e.g., memory and executive functions) depend on. The diagram acts as a reminder of the hierarchical order with which domains should be considered during the assessment and analysis process. The diagram should be read from the bottom level of the gray border upward. For instance, the bottom level of the gray border represents the first factors that need to be considered prior to starting a formal assessment (i.e., What is the patient's level of alertness?; Is he or she oriented?). If the patient has an altered state of consciousness (e.g., delirium or PTA), it is likely that this will mediate performance in all other domains; therefore, the validity of the results on assessment tools designed to measure higher-level functions (e.g., memory, executive functions) would be questionable. In other words, failure on these tests (i.e., memory or tests of executive functioning) may simply represent the patient's acute medical condition (e.g., delirium causing impaired focused attention and thus impaired performance on memory tests) rather than a true organic impairment in a specific cognition function (e.g., memory).

Assuming the examinee is alert and basically oriented, the next factor to consider is whether the examinee has suffered any deficits in his or her senses that might compromise performance on tests that depend on a specific sensory modality. This is illustrated on the diagram by the lower level of the light gray background, which represents the fact that the rest of the core cognitive domains are dependent on intact senses to be assessed accurately. However, where sensory deficits do exist, tests should be selected that minimize the impact of the sensory deficit confounding the results.

When analyzing the results of a neuropsychological assessment, the first level of cognitive abilities to consider are those that are prerequisites for higher-level functions (i.e., attention, processing, and motor speed first, then motor planning, language, and visual abilities). However, if a language impairment (e.g., global aphasia) is suspected, this should be assessed and considered first. Higher-level abilities (e.g., memory and executive functions) should be considered last so that the impact of any deficit in prerequisite skills has been controlled for in the formulation. Most cognitive domains are not pure constructs, they are composites of abilities from several core domains at lower levels of the cognitive functions hierarchy. For instance, working memory is made up of focused attention, short-term memory, and mental flexibility (as illustrated in Figure 5.1 by the items circled with dotted lines). Working memory is a prerequisite to most executive functions, and therefore, despite its name (i.e., "memory"), it is often categorized more as a measure of executive functioning than a measure of memory (hence its position on Figure 5.1 overlapping memory and executive functions). Prospective memory is similarly recognized to be more dependent on executive functions than memory, hence its position on the diagram too. Impaired working memory is usually due to a specific deficit in one of the composite abilities (e.g., impaired mental flexibility); therefore, it is essential to have a good understanding of the cognitive model and which skills are prerequisites for higher-level functions. Misdiagnosis of cognitive deficits can occur when clinicians interpret test scores in isolation without considering whether a deficit in a prerequisite skill is the mediating factor. Correct identification of the underlying cognitive deficit is essential to successful design of cognitive compensatory strategies and NR programs.

On Figure 5.1, the section labeled "current IQ" illustrates that all of the core cognitive domains collectively make up a person's current IQ, and therefore a deficit in any domain should bring into question the validity of a composite IQ score.

During analysis of the assessment measures, the neuropsychologist should be engaging in an iterative process in which an initial hypothesis about the individual's expected performance is formed based on an estimate of the individual's premorbid level of intellectual functioning. The individual's performance on a particular test might prove the neuropsychologist's initial hypothesis false. In this case, the neuropsychologist must form a second hypothesis, based on the new information gathered during the testing of the first hypothesis. This process of progressive hypothesizing continues throughout the analysis of the results. A hypothesis is formed based on one piece of information elicited via the assessment, then compared to the other results to see whether it supports or disproves the hypothesis. The principle of triangulation is employed at this point of the formulation process, to examine similarities and differences within the cognitive profile in accordance with a biopsychosocial model (see Figure 5.2). The

neuropsychological data gathered from the clinical interview, medical investigations, and cognitive test results should correspond (i.e.,
hang together) across the different domains tested (i.e., the biological,
psychological, and social domains).

Results from tests tapping similar cognitive abilities should hang
together, with evidence of the neuroanatomical damage and the functional problems observed. For example, it might be hypothesized that
an individual has a weakness in processing speed following a TBI
because he or she underperforms on a motor task tapping processing speed. To test this hypothesis, the neuropsychologist examines all
other cognitive test results that tap processing speed. If it is an organic
deficit (i.e., related to damage to a specific neuroanatomical region),
processing speed would be expected to be consistently affected across
all timed tasks. In addition, the neuropsychologist might reasonably
expect evidence of neuroanatomical damage consistent with this
result (e.g., reduced GCS at the scene of the accident, PTA lasting
more than 24 hours, and/or an MRI scan indicating diffuse axonal
injury). Poor processing speed might also be expected to be evident
in functional tasks, as described by collateral informants and/or via

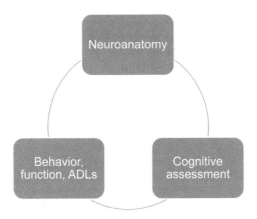

FIGURE 5.2. Triangulation: Data should often correspond across the domains.
Reprinted with permission from Dr. Sanjay Sunak.

self-report measures. However, if the results highlight variability in the individual's performance across the range of tasks tapping processing speed, then the neuropsychologist must generate an alternative hypothesis. In this instance, it might be hypothesized that motor speed is mediating the individual's weaker performance, rather than processing speed. To test this hypothesis the neuropsychologist examines subtests that tap processing speed via a verbal domain, thus excluding the motor component of the task; or examines performance on a pure motor speed task.

Figure 5.3 illustrates the recursive process of progressive hypothesizing that takes place during the analysis of neuropsychological test results. In our experience, this diagram forms a frame of reference to help neuropsychologists hold in mind all the variables they need to consider when analyzing and interpreting standardized test results. If there is inconsistency in the cognitive profile and a lack of triangulation between the biopsychosocial data, this needs to be explained via the neuropsychological formulation (e.g., it may be extraneous factors such as culture, effort, or environmental factors that are hypothesized to be the cause of the patient's presentation).

Failure to conduct neuropsychological formulation in the manner described above can result in erroneous interpretation of cognitive profiles. All too often we have seen neuropsychological assessment reports in which psychologists have interpreted test scores in isolation. This results in misdiagnosis of cognitive dysfunction; for instance, a common error is diagnosing an individual with an auditory memory impairment because of impaired performance on verbal memory tests, when in fact the patient has expressive dysphasia and the memory results have been interpreted without considering them within the context of the individual's impaired performance on a measure of confrontational naming. The starting point of good quality neuropsychological rehabilitation is a sound neuropsychological formulation of the individual's cognitive profile. Figure 5.4 is a formulation sheet developed by Dr. Sanjay Sunak (a clinical neuropsychologist) that we have found is a useful resource to provide to trainee clinical neuropsychologists. It enables them to keep the

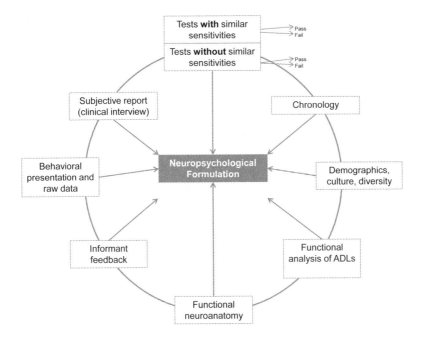

FIGURE 5.3. Neuropsychological assessment formulation framework. Reprinted with permission from Dr. Sanjay Sunak.

core cognitive domains model in mind when formulating a patient's cognitive profile.

Formulation of Neurorehabilitation Needs

The cognition profile is only one aspect taken into consideration when constructing a neuropsychological formulation of a person's rehabilitation needs. A holistic biopsychosocial approach is employed that places the patient at the center and focuses on all aspects of the system around them to help identify the rehabilitation needs. Winegardner and Fish (2017) describe how the process involves inter-disciplinary working to construct a holistic assessment that brings together understanding of the individual's strengths, challenges, and personal identity. In essence, a person-centered and systemic approach is employed to understand the patient's difficulties, rather

ESTIMATED PREMORBID FUNCTION

VCI:	PRI:
WMI:	PSI:
FSIQ:	

CURRENT INTELLECTUAL FUNCTIONING

VCI:	PRI:
WMI:	PSI:
FSIQ:	

EFFORT

PERSONALITY AND COPING STYLE

MOOD

ANXIETY:	DEPRESSION:
PSYCHOSIS:	ADJUSTMENT:

MEMORY

ATTENTION AND WORKING MEMORY

VERBAL:	VISUAL:

NEW LEARNING

VERBAL	VISUAL
ENCODING/ASSIMILATION:	ENCODING/ASSIMILATION:
CONSOLIDATION/RETENTION:	CONSOLIDATION/RETENTION:
RETRIEVAL:	RETRIEVAL:

PROSPECTIVE MEMORY	RETROGRADE AUTOBIOGRAPHICAL MEMORY

VISUAL AND MOTOR SKILLS

VISUAL/MOTOR IMPAIRMENT/MOTOR SPEED:
PERCEPTUAL:
VISUOSPATIAL ORIENTATION/DEPTH PERCEPTION:
VISUOCONSTRUCTION:
PRAXIS:

DEVELOPMENTAL, EDUCATIONAL, AND OCCUPATIONAL HISTORY

LANGUAGE AND HEARING

SEMANTIC:	PHONEMIC:
CONFRONTATIONAL NAMING:	COMPREHENSION:

EXECUTIVE SKILLS

CONCEPTUALIZATION/ABSTRACT REASONING:
DIVIDED ATTENTION/MENTAL FLEXIBILITY:
COGNITIVE SET-SHIFTING/MULTITASKING:
INITIATION/INHIBITION (IMPULSIVITY/PERSEVERATION):
SELECTIVE ATTENTION (RIGIDITY OF THOUGHT):
PLANNING/ORGANIZATION:
PROBLEM SOLVING:
SELF-MONITORING/TIME MANAGEMENT:
SOCIAL PERCEPTION/THEORY OF MIND:

FIGURE 5.4. Neuropsychological assessment formulation sheet. Reprinted with permission from Dr. Sanjay Sunak.

than a traditional medical model, whereby each discipline considers the patient's difficulties from the silo of their own professional perspective of pathology. Using the medical model to formulate fails to take into account the patient's views and premorbid identity, and these aspects can be essential to engagement in rehabilitation. Using neuropsychological formulation, the multidisciplinary assessment results are brought together into a single coherent narrative, which helps the clinician, the team, and the patient to form a shared understanding of the problems.

Presenting this in a visual form helps to summarize information that, in turn, helps to promote a shared understanding and enable unified teamwork (Winson, Wilson, & Bateman, 2017). Once complete, the formulation should lead logically to appropriate interventions. The effectiveness of intervention helps test the formulation and hypotheses, which can be modified if necessary; therefore, the process of progressive hypothesis testing continues throughout rehabilitation. We present here in Figure 5.5 a formulation from the Oliver Zangwill Centre (OZC) in Ely, Cambridgeshire, United Kingdom, to illustrate this process (Winegardner & Fish, 2017).

In our experience, it is essential that the neuropsychological formulation process is conducted transparently and in collaboration with patients, as it facilitates their motivation to engage in the resulting rehabilitation program. This is best illustrated in the words of Jerome Frank (cited by Butler, 1998):

> Patients come to psychotherapy because they are demoralised by the menacing meanings of their symptoms. The therapist collaborates with the patient in formulating a plausible story that makes the meanings of the symptoms more benign and provides procedures for combating them thereby enabling the patient to regain his morale.

The narrative generated via the formulation is drawn upon during rehabilitation to help focus patients on the rationale for aspects of the rehabilitation program that they may be struggling with. The visual diagram of the formulation is shared with the patient and/or

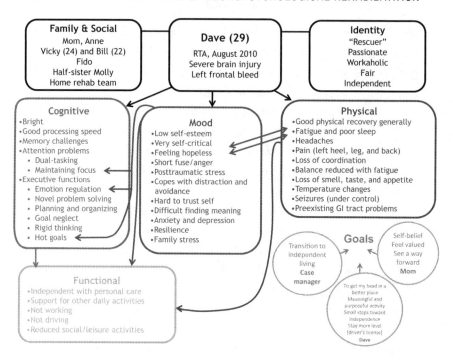

FIGURE 5.5. Holistic formulation framework. Reprinted with permission from the Oliver Zangwill Centre for Neuropsychological Rehabilitation.

their family and updated, along with the goals, as hypotheses are progressively tested and proved or disproved.

We attach here three instruments that may help clinicians plan their assessments. The first (Figure 5.6) is a tool to aid the neuropsychological interview (Kapur & Bradley, 2018). The second (Figure 5.7) is an outline of a clinical interview used at the OZC (Jill Winegardner, personal communication, 2018). The third (Figures 5.8 and 5.9) is a screening tool used with more severely impaired patients at the Raphael Hospital (Anita Rose and Heidi Hand, personal communication, 2018). This has been completed with a patient whose details have been changed and anonymized.

It is hoped that these instruments will provide guidance in thinking about the questions we need to ask in order to understand the problems faced by our patients and help decide which goals are important to them.

CLINICAL DETAILS	Medical screening: Cardiac, blood pressure, cholesterol, smoking.	Neurological screening: Birth/milestones, head injury, epilepsy, loss of consciousness, funny turns. Check for ictal/postictal amnesia.	COGNITION, EMOTION, AND MOTIVATION		Concentration: Gives up or is distracted easily. Daydreams. Difficulty driving and talking. Flips between tasks. Falls asleep watching TV. Mind wanders during reading, group conversation. Goes off on a tangent in a conversation.		Speech: Word-finding—high-frequency words, getting stuck, OR word substitutions, transient. Returns after a while or with cues. Mispronounces words. Speech comprehension.
Sleep, tiredness.	Psychiatric screening: Taken antidepressants, seen psychiatrist. Recent stressful life events, family history.	Family history of neurological disease	Current medication				
Family setting and adjustment. Social--friends.							
Change in food preferences. Alcohol abuse, illicit drugs.	Memory--frequency, severity, change.	Repeatedly asks what day it is	Repeats him/herself three or more times a day, most days.	Where items are kept at home, supermarket.	Memory difficulties when reading books or watching TV.		
Headache, backache, stomachache	Forgets deaths of family/friends, pets, people in news. Forgets holidays.	Forgets messages. Forgets appointments. Forgets to take medication.	Uncharacteristic difficulty in learning new gadgets/pieces of equipment.	Navigation problems—way back to, within hotel if on vacation. After shopping--finding car.	Due to memory, cannot now do things did before--ADLs, job, hobbies, DIY.		Other language: Reading, writing, spelling.
INSTRUMENTAL ACTIVITIES OF DAILY LIVING AND EXECUTIVE FUNCTION	Hobbies, interests, music, sports, achievements, vacations. Media exposure (TV, radio, papers, Internet).		Education--best / worst subjects, number of exams passed, reading/writing problems.				Vision, hearing, etc. Double vision.
	Occupation (first, best, last) Premorbid strengths / weaknesses						Visual neglect.
	Medical and psychiatric history	Family history			R–L hand	Reading glasses	Smell, taste, libido.
Occupational adjustment	Early symptoms: Frequency during the day:	Duration:	Change over time: Frequency during the week (e.g., daily?):				Calculating skill
Technical, dealing with people, stressful events. Learning new routines, evidence from superiors or colleagues.	Purpose is to probe memory, to assess speech, and to build rapport. With outpatient, when did you leave home? With inpatient, when were you admitted, tests, visitors? Start off with general conversation about hobbies/sports, vacations, tests, treatment (including medication), and TV. Ask who, when, where questions. See below for further questions. *** Purpose of assessment (reason for referral). Nature of assessment (cognitive, not psychiatric). Test procedures (what's involved, time to prepare and score). How patient feels about testing. Use of information (clinical, audit, etc.). Confidentiality (who will get information). Feedback (when given, patient gets copy of report). Home situation. If recording, consent to record.						Reality distortion: Hallucinations/confabulation. "Eyes or ears play tricks..." (things, people, animals). Delusions.
Mental slowing. Making decisions. Planning. Dealing with problems.							Depression: Feels sad. Libido down. Seldom laughs. Eating/drinking change. Sleep disturbed. Suicidal. Indecisive about past, future. Tearful. A.M. worse. Lost interest in pastimes, leisure, and appearance.
Driving and related: Accidents/near accidents. Recall of parked car. Navigating familiar and unfamiliar routes. Use of satnav.							
Cooking and for several people. Leaves equipment on.							Motivation: Past hobbies/pastimes. Hygiene, cleanliness. Change of clothes. Eating.
Change in ability to use TV, DIY equipment, kitchen appliances.							Tolerance level: Verbal—anger. Physical—aggression.
Make/answer phone calls. Use all features of mobile phone.							Anxiety: Panic attacks. Chronic anxiety.
Use of computer, Internet, email.							Disinhibition: Verbal, social, financial, toilet, sexual.
Shopping in stores and online. Handling coins. Dealing with bills, bank accounts.							Obsessionality/ stereotyped behavior: Obsessional thinking/ruminations.
Eating habits and preferences. Table manners.							Emotional lability: Spontaneous or triggered by event.
Bath, shower, shave, make-up.							*Worried Well –* What it is not--fatal, "mad." Genuine--not making up, common, "functional."
Dressing--ability, appropriate.	IN THE CASE OF THOSE WHO HAVE LIMITED FLUENCY IN ENGLISH, OR HAVE MINIMAL EDUCATION OR ARE FROM ANOTHER CULTURE, TRY TO GET INFORMATION FROM ONE OR TWO INFORMANTS.						
Lacks judgment when buying items, responding to offers, gambling.	*** 1. Doctors seen before--names, when, content. Drug history--what, when.	2. What had for supper yesterday evening. Tests, scans, etc.--when and A.M./P.M., who else was there.	3. Recent vacations/trips-- when, incidents/events from episode or journey to/from.	4. Ages--self, spouse, children, grandchildren (and names).	5. Day, month, year (date).		Reversible. Because brain is physically intact, things can be done to help.
Any activities spouse has had to do over.	6. Provide names of personalities who have died--ask if familiar, and for details. Note media exposure-- Mohammad Ali, Nelson Mandela, Michael Jackson, Osama Bin Laden, Saddam Hussein.						Effects of fatigue, stress, hypervigilance, pain. How states of mind > physical symptoms.
Coping on vacations	7. Reading books--ask for title, author, content of current book or last one read. TV program recently watched.						
	8. U.K. Prime Minister, Leader of Opposition, U.S. President, Queen Elizabeth's children. Prince Charles's wife and children.						Software-hardware, car / piano out of tune.
After poor performance, ask about concentration during testing	9. U.K. Prime Ministers and U.S. Presidents in recent years; Royal family members; current London mayor.						
	MALINGERING--I. If appropriate, warn before-hand about need for maximum effort and that poor effort can be detected. Establish good rapport. Bad news: some scores very low. Good	MALINGERING--II. Perhaps due to the stress he/she is going through; some find it difficult to be fully engaged and to stay motivated during testing, and this can affect their concentration and the amount of effort		Anger--**S.T.O.P.** Stop. Think. Other Perspectives.			*Problem Solving--* **S.T.O.P.** Stop Think
	news: low scores due to non-neurological treatable factors.	they put into a test. Ask patient, Do you think this applied in your case?		Other Possible actions. Refrain, Reframe, Remove mentally/physically from situation.			*Organize--what to do* **Plan--**when, how

Say to the patient he/she has "done well," to be patient, positive, persevere. Encourage him/her to accept, adapt to, embrace, and show self-compassion to situation. Cognitive reframing, humor, support groups/organizations, adjust goals and expectations. Spiritual or charitable activities, meditation--these need to be advised as appropriate, and with sensitivity to individual and context.

FIGURE 5.6. Neuropsychological Interview. From Kapur and Bradley (2018). Reprinted with permission from Narinder Kapur and Veronica Bradley, London Neuropsychology Clinic.

IDENTIFYING INFORMATION

Name _____ Sex _____

Date seen _____ Age _____ Date of birth _____

Handedness _____ Address _____

Telephone contact person _____

Referral source _____

Referral source contact information _____

OBSERVATIONS

❑ Contact telephone
❑ General appearance
❑ Ability to manage details of program participation
❑ Social interactions

MEDICAL INFORMATION

❑ Date of injury
❑ Diagnosis
❑ History of injury
❑ Medical information
❑ Medical history
❑ Psychiatric history
❑ Drug and alcohol use
❑ Current medications

SOCIAL HISTORY

❑ Where born and raised
❑ Education—grade completed and grades/learning problems/special needs/above average
❑ Work history—include type of work, responsibilities, quality of performance, regularity
❑ Legal history
❑ Military history
❑ Family–marital status, children, lives with whom?
❑ Social networks—both before and after injury
❑ Leisure interests/hobbies/sports—both before and after injury

PRESENTING COMPLAINTS

Physical

❑ Weakness
❑ Balance
❑ Dizziness
❑ Headache
❑ Fatigue
❑ Vision changes
❑ Hearing changes

❑ Changes in touch, taste, or smell
❑ Temperature dysregulation

Cognitive

❑ General intellectual ability
❑ Orientation
❑ Attention and concentration
❑ Learning and memory
❑ Visual processing
❑ Language and communication
❑ Social cognition
❑ Executive dysfunction
❑ Metacognition (awareness of self in relation to others and the world around him or her, theory of mind)

Mood/emotions

❑ Depression
❑ Grief
❑ Anxiety, including obsessive–compulsive behaviors
❑ Posttraumatic stress
❑ Irritability/anger
❑ Emotional dyscontrol
❑ Interpersonal interactions
❑ Self-esteem and self-confidence
❑ Identity

Social

❑ Family
❑ Friends
❑ School or work
❑ Groups (religious, charity work, clubs, sports)

Functional skills

❑ Basic ADLs (bathing, dressing, grooming, hygiene, toileting)
❑ Domestic ADLs (laundry, shopping, cooking, money management including banking, transportation including driving)
❑ Leisure and recreation
❑ School
❑ Volunteer work
❑ Competitive employment

FIGURE 5.7. Checklist for initial interview. Reprinted with permission from Jill Winegardner, Oliver Zangwill Centre for Neuropsychological Rehabilitation.

Patient: Derek Montague Rose **Preferred Name:** Monty	**Age on Admission:** 46 **Date of Birth:** August 17, 1972 **Gender:** Male
Address: xxx	**Next of Kin:** Josie Rose **Relationship:** Wife **Contact Number:** xxx
Date Admitted: February 6, 2018 **Funding body:** xxx CCG; Level 2a	**Admitted from:** Ward 2, Hospital xxx **Handover Available/Received?** Yes—discharge report and therapists' reports
Handedness: Right **Glasses?** No **Hearing Aid?** No	**First Language:** English **Nationality:** British

MEDICAL HISTORY	
Presenting Diagnosis: TBI following RTA. Subsequent subarachnoid hemorrhage and subdural hematoma.	**Date of Injury:** April 1, 2018

History of Injury/Description (including scans): RTA—pedestrian hit by car. Sustained traumatic brain injury with SAH, SDH, and skull fractures, and mild dissection of right internal carotid artery (+ non-brain-related injuries).

Initial report of seizures on arrival at A&E; however, no episodes of seizures since.

MRI indicated frontal contusions, SAH, and SDH in temporal and parietal lobes. No midline shift. Ventricles normal.

Previous Treating Facilities for This Injury: While at the xxxx Hospital, Mr. Rose received multiple interventions for brain injury, including bifrontal decompressive craniotomy due to rising ICPs (April 5, 2018) and craniotomy insertion (June 5, 2018).

(continued)

FIGURE 5.8. Example of a completed Raphael Hospital Department of Neuropsychology Admission Psychology Screen. The patient's identifying details have been disguised. Reprinted with permission from Anita Rose and Heidi Hand.

Current Medications:	

Relevant Previous Medical History/Family Medical History: *Nothing of note.*	

PSYCHOSOCIAL HISTORY	
Family and Nature of Relationships: *Wife, two children—son and daughter, three siblings, parents, and in-laws. All very supportive.*	**Other Social Support:** *Colleagues at the church in which he is employed. Large social network.*
Previous Living Arrangements: *Owns home, lives with wife and children.*	**Hobbies and Activities:** *Soccer (supports local team) socializing with his family and friends. Religion is very important to Monty.*
Employment History *(including current work situation):* *Works as office manager at local church.*	**Educational History** *(including age left education, any learning needs and qualifications): GCSEs, BTEc, and theology training.*
Previous Mental Health Concerns: *None of note.*	**Previous Contact with Mental Health Services or Professionals** *(dates/purpose): None.*
Substance Use History: *None.*	**Other Significant Life Events/ Relevant Information** *(losses, trauma, etc.): None.*
CURRENT PRESENTATION	
Level of Awareness *(if applicable):* *Monty is aware of his physical difficulties and his memory problems; however, he has a low awareness of his other current cognitive difficulties (attention, impulsivity, visual neglect) that are placing him at risk.*	**Physical Status** *(transfers/ mobility): Fully mobile although can be a little impulsive at times and is easily distracted. It is also noted that he "misses" doorways, steps, and is unsafe on stairs.*
Continence Status: *Fully continent.*	**Feeding/Swallowing Status:** *Normal diet.*
Language/Communication: *No concerns around Communication.*	**Other Relevant Information:** *Nothing of note.*

FIGURE 5.8. *(continued)*

COGNITION	
Preadmission Reported Cognitive Impairments: *Cognitive deficits reported, mainly memory and possible visual neglect (no record of side).*	**Previous Neuropsychological Assessments:** *None recorded and no evidence of previous assessments.*
Patient Self-Reported Cognitive Difficulties: *He reports some memory problems with recent events and given information. Appears unaware of visual problems, attention difficulties. or impulsivity.*	**Relevant Team Observations:** <u>Physiotherapy</u>: *Participation is good, motivated to engage, unsafe on stairs due to cognitive problems and visual neglect.* <u>Occupational therapy</u>: *Main deficits noted include attention and memory. Did not want to engage in cooking tasks, reporting wife completes all housework tasks.*
Cognitive Screen/Assessment of Orientation: *On admission MOCA 22/30. Oriented to place but not to time and date.*	**Relevant Family Observations:** *Wife reports no real changes in personality or behavior but is concerned with regard to his memory.*

Initial Formulation/Summary:
Monty has some awareness of his cognitive difficulties; however, he appears unaware of deficits that have been reported to place him at risk. He is reported to be willing to engage and to be motivated in therapy input. He is willing to undergo assessment and has agreed to join the Brain Injury Awareness Group. He is concerned around returning to work although believes that "God" will support him.

PLAN FOR ONGOING PSYCHOLOGICAL INPUT:
Monty will attend the Brain Injury Awareness Group; this will support in increasing his understanding of the biopsychosocial effects of his brain injury, in a peer-supported environment. A comprehensive neuropsychological assessment will be commenced with immediate effect. An orientation protocol will be put in place and his keyworkers trained in administration.

Any Immediate Protocol Required (e.g., orientation, confabulation):
YES—orientation   *Date completed:*
                                                      DOA

BEHAVIOR	
Preadmission Behavioral Presentation: *No concerns.*	**Preadmission Behavioral Management Strategies:** *N/A.*

Behavioral Presentation Since Admission (ABCs, initial observations, interdisciplinary notes, etc.): *No concerns raised.*

FIGURE 5.8. (*continued*)

Initial Formulation/Summary: *Monty does not present with any behavioral concerns.*

PLAN FOR ONGOING PSYCHOLOGICAL INPUT: *No input required currently with regard to behavioral issues.*

Behavioral care plan required? *No*	*Date completed:*
Behavioral guidelines/protocols required? *No*	*Date completed:*
Monitoring charts required *No*	*Date completed:*
Functional behavioral analysis required? *No*	*Date completed:*
Positive behavioral support plan required? *No*	*Date completed:*

EMOTIONAL WELL-BEING

Self-Reported Current Mood *(e.g., feeling low/depressed, anxiety, angry, suicide/self-harm risks, flashbacks/PTSD):* *Monty reports feeling "OK." He reports no concerns with regard to his emotional well-being.*

Self-Reported Previous Mental Health Concerns: *None.*

Self-Reported Coping Strategies (past and present): *His faith is very important and provides all his needs to cope with challenges in life. Believes prayer and support from his family and friends provide structure and help him cope.*

Relevant Interdisciplinary Reports/Observations *(e.g., withdrawal, avoidance, aggression, agitation, anxiety, hallucinations, distress):* *No concerns raised.*

Mood Screens Administered and Results *(HADS, DISCS, DASS, BASDECs, BDI, BAI, STAI):* *HADS administered—all within normal parameters.*

Risk of Self-Harm or Suicide: *None.*

FIGURE 5.8. *(continued)*

Initial Formulation and Summary: *Monty's reports his emotional well-being as stable. This concurs with reports of family and staff. There is no reported premorbid mental health history or concerns around his psychological status. His faith is a protective factor.*

PLAN FOR ONGOING PSYCHOLOGICAL INPUT: *Currently there is no concern around his emotional well-being; however, he will remain under the monitoring system.*

Nursing/Emotional Well-Being Care Plan in Place? *Yes—as standard on admission.*   *Date completed: DOA*

Suicide Risk Assessment Required? *No*

Date completed:

OVERALL SUMMARY

Initial Formulation and Summary: *Monty sustained a TBI on April 1, 2018—he is approximately 8 weeks postinjury. He has made a good physical recovery. There are no concerns around changes in personality and behavior. He reports positive emotional well-being and to date no concerns have been raised. He has some awareness of his cognitive difficulties, namely, memory; however, he appears unaware of the noted attentional problems and visual neglect. He has been noted to be impulsive at times, placing him at risk in certain situations such as on stairs. He is disoriented to time and date. His faith is very important, as is his family and social network. These will provide supportive structure to his rehabilitation.*

Patient Goals: *To improve memory.*
To return to work.

PLAN FOR ONGOING PSYCHOLOGICAL INPUT: *Full neuropsychological assessment to be completed and subsequent neurorehabilitation to be planned following results.*
Visual neglect assessment and possible intervention—priority.
Monty is to attend the Brain Injury Awareness Group.

Actions: *Orientation Program*
Neuropsychological Assessment
Neglect Assessment
Brain Injury Awareness Group and 1:1 Sessions for Brain Injury Awareness
Refer to Chaplaincy Team
Place on Monitoring System of Emotional Well-Being
Vocational Support

Psychological Input Status:
Active
Monitoring
Closed

A COPY OF THIS SCREEN IS TO BE PLACED IN THE PATIENT'S FILE AND PROVIDED TO THE PATIENT (if appropriate).

FIGURE 5.8. (*continued*)

Patient:	Age on Admission:
Preferred Name:	Date of Birth:
	Gender:
Address:	Next of Kin:
	Relationship:
	Contact Number:
Date Admitted:	Admitted from:
Funding body:	
	Handover Available/Received?
Handedness:	First Language:
Glasses?	Nationality:
Hearing Aid?	

MEDICAL HISTORY	
Presenting Diagnosis:	Date of Injury:

History of Injury/Description (including scans):

Previous Treating Facilities for This Injury:

(continued)

FIGURE 5.9. Raphael Hospital Department of Neuropsychology Admission Psychology Screen. Reprinted with permission from Anita Rose and Heidi Hand.

From *Essentials of Neuropsychological Rehabilitation* by Barbara A. Wilson and Shai Betteridge. Copyright © 2019 The Guilford Press. Permission to photocopy this figure is granted to purchasers of this book for personal use or use with individual patients (see copyright page for details). Purchasers can download and print enlarged versions of this figure (see the box at the end of the table of contents).

Current Medications:

Relevant Previous Medical History/Family Medical History:

PSYCHOSOCIAL HISTORY	
Family and Nature of Relationships:	Other Social Support:
Previous Living Arrangements:	Hobbies and Activities:
Employment History *(including current work situation)*:	Educational History *(including age left education, any learning needs and qualifications)*:
Previous Mental Health Concerns:	Previous Contact with Mental Health Services or Professionals *(dates/purpose)*:
Substance Use History:	Other Significant Life Events/ Relevant Information *(losses, trauma, etc.)*:
CURRENT PRESENTATION	
Level of Awareness *(if applicable)*:	Physical Status *(transfers/ mobility)*:
Continence Status:	Feeding/Swallowing Status:
Language/Communication:	Other Relevant Information:

FIGURE 5.9. *(continued)*

COGNITION	
Preadmission Reported Cognitive Impairments:	**Previous Neuropsychological Assessments:**
Patient Self-Reported Cognitive Difficulties:	**Relevant Team Observations:**
Cognitive Screen/Assessment of Orientation:	**Relevant Family Observations:**
Initial Formulation/Summary:	
PLAN FOR ONGOING PSYCHOLOGICAL INPUT:	

Any Immediate Protocol Required *(e.g., orientation, confabulation):*
                                    Date completed:
                                    DOA	

BEHAVIOR	
Preadmission Behavioral Presentation:	**Preadmission Behavioral Management Strategies:**
Behavioral Presentation Since Admission *(ABCs, initial observations, interdisciplinary notes, etc.):*	

FIGURE 5.9. *(continued)*

Initial Formulation/Summary:
PLAN FOR ONGOING PSYCHOLOGICAL INPUT:
Behavioral care plan required? *Date completed:*
Behavioral guidelines/protocols required? *Date completed:*
Monitoring charts required *Date completed:*
Functional behavioral analysis required? *Date completed:*
Positive behavioral support plan required? *Date completed:*
EMOTIONAL WELL-BEING
Self-Reported Current Mood *(e.g., feeling low/depressed, anxiety, angry, suicide/self-harm risks, flashbacks/PTSD):*
Self-Reported Previous Mental Health Concerns:
Self-Reported Coping Strategies (past and present):
Relevant Interdisciplinary Reports/Observations *(e.g., withdrawal, avoidance, aggression, agitation, anxiety, hallucinations, distress):*
Mood Screens Administered and Results *(HADS, DISCS, DASS, BASDECs, BDI, BAI, STAI):*
Risk of Self-Harm or Suicide:

FIGURE 5.9. (*continued*)

Initial Formulation and Summary:

PLAN FOR ONGOING PSYCHOLOGICAL INPUT:

Nursing/Emotional Well-Being Care Plan in Place?	
	Date completed: DOA

Suicide Risk Assessment Required?	
	Date completed:

OVERALL SUMMARY

Initial Formulation and Summary:

Patient Goals:

PLAN FOR ONGOING PSYCHOLOGICAL INPUT:

Actions:

Psychological Input Status: *Active* *Monitoring* *Closed*

A COPY OF THIS SCREEN IS TO BE PLACED IN THE PATIENT'S FILE AND PROVIDED TO THE PATIENT (if appropriate).

FIGURE 5.9. (*continued*)

102

CHAPTER 6

The Need for a Working Partnership in Neuropsychological Rehabilitation

Introduction

In former times, doctors, psychologists, therapists, and other involved professionals would decide what a patient should focus on, aim for, or work toward in rehabilitation. They might have concluded by suggesting that the client and the therapist would work toward wheelchair independence for the client, or the introduction of an alternative communication system. Whatever decision was made, the patient would have no say in the matter. Now, in the 21st century, it is recognized by most professionals working in rehabilitation that their work consists of a partnership between patients, families, and health care staff, who share with each other in making decisions as to how to proceed in the rehabilitation process.

What Do We Mean by a "Partnership"?

Wilson (2003b) suggested that "rehabilitation is now seen as a partnership between people with brain injury, their families/carers and health service staff" (p. 294). Such a partnership relies upon a shared understanding between the patient/client, family, clinical team, and any others involved in the care of the person with a brain injury. Kate, a patient known to one of us (Wilson), requested help in working together (Wilson & Bainbridge, 2014). She was severely physically disabled following encephalitis caused by an autoimmune response and had a caregiver come to her home every day to carry out intimate tasks such as giving her regular enemas. Importantly, Kate requested help in persuading her caregivers to treat her as a person and not a mere body. Other patients who participated in decision making included Sonia, who had survived a gunshot wound to the head and wanted to be able to cook a meal for her friends; Martin, who had sustained a mild stroke and needed to understand what had happened to him; and Peter, who had survived a TBI and wanted to look after his children while his wife went to work. For a detailed discussion of the ways these and other brain-injured patients work in partnership with rehabilitation staff, see Wilson et al. (2014).

As far back as 1986, Prigatano et al. argued that a working alliance is "crucial for shifting the patient from being a dependent, convalescing person to being a more fully functioning, independent individual" (p. 155). Such an alliance can also be achieved by collaboration between all people involved in the rehabilitation process, consisting of regular meetings with families and all team members and groups comprising ex-clients who provide input and advice to present users. Examples of collaboration in our own work include partnerships with employers and college staff for people who wish to return to work or further education. We have worked with a university lecturer to help a young woman obtain a PhD in mathematics after she sustained a brain injury, and we have also worked with college tutors to help a music student return to her studies.

One of our most successful clients at the OZC was Mark, who held a senior position in a firm of insurance underwriters prior to a severe TBI while on a mountain biking vacation in Switzerland (Wilson & Palmer, 2014). He was airlifted to a specialist hospital where he was found to have a severe brain injury. He was in a coma for a week and in PTA for another week. A CT scan showed a diffuse axonal injury, edema, small deep midline hemorrhages, and a subdural hematoma. He developed meningitis, pneumonia, and septicemia. Eventually, he stabilized and was transferred back to London, where he lived. He came to the OZC 9 months postinjury. He was referred for help with memory, attention, and planning problems. Mark was described as lacking initiative. He had some insight but did not appreciate the nature and extent of his memory problems nor the potential impact of these on his work.

When assessed by us, we found that his intellectual functioning was above average but he had particular problems with memory being below the first percentile on a well-known memory test. He also had some executive deficits with planning and organization.

Mark had expected our team would say he could return to work. If he had returned he would almost certainly have failed to hold down his job and would probably have been labeled as unemployable in a demanding field. Instead, he entered our program where his goals were to:

1. Develop an awareness of his strengths and weaknesses in a written form.
2. Describe how these would impact his domestic, social, and work situations.
3. Identify whether he could return to his former employment (underwriter for an insurance company).
4. Manage his own financial affairs independently.
5. Demonstrate competence in negotiating skills, as rated by a work colleague.
6. Develop a range of leisure interests.

Although Mark attended groups and had individual sessions like all our other clients, it is his return to work that we focus on here to illustrate the partnership with Mark's employers. The early work was done at the OZC: through attendance at the memory group and individual memory work, Mark began to use a diary for appointments and things to do. He then started to use a computer "contacts" card for recording relevant information (such as the birthday of his boss's child). He soon adapted mnemonic strategies to learn people's names and other information and then developed a database for high-risk areas such as where earthquakes were likely to happen or where there had been an oil spill (as these kinds of events would affect whether or not a business would be insured). Then came the beginning of Mark's return to work. His employers worked closely with the team, advising us on the tasks Mark would need to master. Mark then went to work 1 day a week. At first he shadowed a colleague, then he began to deal with minimal-risk situations supervised by another employee. He then stepped up to 2 days a week with a gradual step-by-step increase in his responsibilities. These steps allowed his manager to develop confidence in Mark's judgment in a high-risk business. It also enabled Mark to develop his own confidence as well as allowing time for him to learn to apply the strategies he had been introduced to at the OZC.

Seven months after starting the program, Mark was reinstated on the company payroll at full salary. Several years later he remains employed and indeed has been head-hunted (contacted by other companies to leave his present employer and join them) several times. He is married with two daughters and helps to run a cycling club for youngsters. He feels his memory is not as good as it should be, so he still uses his diary, mnemonics, and other strategies he learned at the OZC. By working he contributes to the cost of his rehabilitation through the taxes he pays (his employer also pays taxes). Mark has never claimed or received welfare benefits, so intensive rehabilitation in this case was clinically and economically effective. The collaboration with his employer was successful.

To illustrate partnership with a patient, his wife's family, and with university students (employed to provide support following rehabilitation), we report now the case of EO, a 64-year-old man who had survived autoimmune limbic encephalitis in April 2013. This had left him severely amnesic. He was referred to us in 2015 for help with the cognitive and emotional consequences of his memory impairments (Fish, Pamment, & Brentnall, 2017). The primary interventions implemented were "attention process training" (Sohlberg & Mateer, 1989), use of NeuroPage alerts to remind EO to check his diary (Wilson et al., 2001), errorless learning to teach EO how to use Google maps (Wilson et al., 1994), and family support. Following successful rehabilitation, we realized that after discharge EO would need support at home to help with his daily diary planning. Together with EO and his wife, it was decided to enlist three psychology students from a local university. The university helped identify volunteers. EO and his wife were heavily involved in the selection and recruitment process. Three volunteers were recruited, and entered the program with commitment and enthusiasm, each committing to 3–4 hours per week over one to two mornings for a minimum of 6 months. In exchange, they gained learning opportunities, practical experience relevant to clinical psychology, and accessed supervision from a health professional. Outcomes from this partnership were very positive, as EO participated in a wider range of community activities including sitting on a board of governors at a local school, listening to children reading, and attending an archaeology club. On formal measures, there was a 22% reduction in severity of overall symptoms as measured by the EBIQ (Teasdale et al., 1997), a 27% reduction in dysexecutive symptoms as measured by the Dyexecutive Questionnaire—Revised (Simblett et al., 2017), and a 43% reduction in carer burden as measured by the Modified Care Giver Strain Index (Thornton & Travis, 2003).

There were qualitative benefits too, with one of the students saying, "This role has reinforced my love for psychology (and helping people), and I now feel I have matured and would be better prepared for any clinical work in the future." Another said, "This role has helped me have a new understanding of neurological deficits and the effects it has on someone's life, and has helped me greatly improve my interpersonal skills and grow as a person. . . . It was extremely rewarding and I enjoyed it thoroughly." EO himself commented, "I am grateful for the support of the OZC, along with that received from the Encephalitis Society, and most importantly from my family. My life has changed forever, but I am embracing the new life and now look forward and not backward—as backward I cannot remember anyway!" His wife of 45 years said, "Once the girls [i.e., the volunteers] came in, I could switch off and know that E. was in good hands. It allows me to stay as wife, not a carer" (Fish et al., 2017).

Klonoff et al. (2017) remind us of the importance of including family members in the process of neuropsychological rehabilitation, as this maximizes awareness, acceptance, and realism about the injury. It also reduces suffering and cultivates coping, adaptability, growth, and optimism. Prince (2017) also stresses the importance of family work. Ylvisaker and Feeney (2000) stressed that rehabilitation needs to involve personally meaningful themes, activities, settings, and interactions. Tate, Strettles, and Osoteo (2003) also implied, by the very nature of their work, the importance of partnership in the descriptions of their service for people with brain injury. These ways of regarding rehabilitation require that people with brain injury, rehabilitation staff, and others work together and, furthermore, work on what is important for brain-injured people and their families.

All too often in the past, and to a large extent in some practices today, clients or patients (we use these terms interchangeably) in rehabilitation work on exercises or tasks that do not help to reduce their everyday problems. It cannot be emphasized enough that this is not what rehabilitation is about. While individual patients may improve on the tasks they practice, such practice rarely generalizes to the real-life problems they face. There is no strong evidence that brain training actually reduces real-life problems (Max Planck Institute for Human Development and Stanford Center on Longevity, 2014). A special issue on brain training in the journal *Neuropsychological Rehabilitation*, edited by van Heugten, Kessels, and Ponds, appeared in 2016. The editors contributed an article entitled "Brain Training: Hype or Hope?" In an editorial, they wrote that "brain training is topical yet controversial. Effects are often limited to trained tasks; and near and far effects to untrained tasks or everyday measures are often small or lacking altogether" (p. 639). The editors also say that future studies should include outcome measures on daily functioning, self-efficacy, and quality of life (Van Heugten et al., 2016).

We now look at some group studies involving the principle of working together followed by a presentation of individual cases that illustrate the principles of partnership.

Examples of Working Together in Clinical Practice

Group Studies: NeuroPage

One of the best-evaluated technological aids for helping people with memory and/or executive deficits to cope in everyday life is NeuroPage, a system whereby messages are sent out, using a pager or text message via a mobile phone, to help survivors of brain injury compensate for everyday memory and planning problems. NeuroPage was developed by a neuropsychologist, Neil Hersch, working together with Larry Treadgold, the engineer father of a young man who sustained a severe traumatic brain injury (Hersch & Treadgold, 1999).

Evaluation of NeuroPage in the United Kingdom began in 1994. The results show that not only are these studies an example of how research can influence clinical practice, they are also a good example of partnership between researchers, health care staff, people with brain injury, and their families. Each participant to be included in the study was interviewed by a member of the staff working on the NeuroPage project in the presence of one or more family members or therapists working with the brain-injured person. A discussion followed about the kinds of things the person needed or wanted to remember in order to be more independent. A test message (e.g., "Please open the window") was sent on the pager to see if the person could respond appropriately. This was all the training required. A list of messages, usually agreed to by all parties, was drawn up, with the person having the problems being given the final say, and on occasions overriding the message the family member wanted. The wording of the reminder message was also decided by the brain-injured person. Some wanted the messages to be as short as possible (such as "Get up") while others chose something longer (such as "Good morning, X, it is time to get up"). Typically, between four and seven messages were sent each day, although there could be far more or even less depending on the person's needs.

The first trial was a pilot study (Wilson, Evans, Emslie, & Malinek, 1997), which involved 15 people. Each client selected target behaviors they wanted to remember each day (e.g., "Take your medication"; "Don't forget your hearing aid"; "Catch the 8:40 bus"). During a 6-week baseline phase, independent observers (usually relatives) monitored whether or not the targets had been achieved.

Clients were then provided with NeuroPage for 12 weeks. The pager reminded them of the target behaviors, and these were monitored, as before in the baseline phase. Following the treatment phase, clients returned their pagers and were monitored for a further 4 weeks. The group as a whole improved from a success rate of 37% in the baseline phase to over 85% in the treatment phase. Furthermore, every one of the 15 clients showed a statistically significant improvement between baseline and treatment. When the pagers were returned, performance for the group as a whole fell slightly to 74%, which still represented a considerable improvement over baseline (Wilson et al., 1997). Two single-case studies demonstrated that NeuroPage was able to increase independence (Evans, Emslie, & Wilson, 1998; Wilson et al., 1999), and a randomized controlled trial, in which 143 patients completed all stages of the trial, was published in 2001 (Wilson et al., 2001). Anyone was accepted into the trial if they felt they needed the service, could read the message on the screen, and could respond appropriately to the test message. We were not selective. The youngest participant was 8 years old and the oldest 73. We included several different diagnoses. Following a 2-week baseline period, clients were randomly allocated to pager first group or waiting list first group. After 7 weeks with NeuroPage or 7 weeks on the waiting list, those with the pager returned it and those on the waiting list received a pager. Targets were monitored as described in the pilot study. Over 80% of the clients were more successful in achieving their everyday targets in the pager period than in the baseline period.

Until recently, the randomized controlled trial of NeuroPage was the only such trial to be carried out with electronic aids and it is still the largest trial conducted (De Joode, van Heugten, Verhey, & van Boxtel, 2010). As a result of the trial, the local health service set up a NeuroPage service for people throughout the United Kingdom (Wilson, Scott, Evans, & Emslie, 2003; Saez, Deakins, Winson, Watson, & Wilson, 2011). Some people required the reminder service for years but the average length of time for each individual was 6 months, as most people learned their routines within this period. All messages were, of course, chosen by the person with the problems. Since 2007, people can choose to have messages sent to a mobile phone if preferred.

A Series of Single-Case Studies: People with Alzheimer's Disease

A series of papers by Clare et al. between 1999 and 2002, showed that people with Alzheimer's disease could learn useful everyday information when errorless learning, spaced retrieval, and vanishing cues were combined. Errorless learning and spaced retrieval were discussed in the previous chapter. Vanishing cues is another method employed in memory rehabilitation for helping memory-impaired people to learn more efficiently. First described by Glisky, Schacter, and Tulving (1986), this is a method whereby prompts are provided and then gradually faded. For example, someone learning a new name might be expected first to copy the whole name, then the last letter would be deleted, the name would be copied again and the last letter inserted, then the last two letters would be deleted and the process repeated until all letters were completed by the person learning the name. In the first study, Clare, Wilson, Breen, and Hodges (1999) were able to teach VJ, a 74-year-old man in the early stages of Alzheimer's disease, the names of his colleagues at his lawn bowls club. These names were those that VJ himself wanted to relearn. Following the principle of errorless learning, preventing errors as far as possible, they used a combination of strategies, which included finding a distinctive feature of the face, vanishing cues, and spaced retrieval. For example, one of the people at the club was named Carol, and her name was learned using a combination of all the methods described above. The distinctive feature selected was her curl, which VJ was asked to associate with the name (Carol with the curl). At the same time, vanishing cues was employed so that VJ was given written versions of the name with progressively more letters omitted, as in the following example: CAROL, CARO_, CAR__, and so on. VJ completed the missing letters and eventually learned the name without any cues. These two strategies were combined with spaced retrieval (otherwise known as expanded rehearsal). VJ learned the names of his colleagues using photographs in his memory therapy sessions, and demonstrated generalization by greeting his colleagues by name at the lawn bowls club. A similar study with another man with Alzheimer's disease showed similar results (Clare, Wilson, Carter, Roth, & Hodges, 2002). Much of this work was completed as part of Clare's PhD dissertation (Clare, 2000). All the people with Alzheimer's disease chose what they wanted to work on and all selected things important in their everyday lives, which included relearning the names of grandchildren; relearning how to tell the time, and relearning how to recognize coins again. One woman wanted to learn to check a memory board so that she did not irritate her husband by repeatedly asking him the same question. Much of this work is summarized in a book by Clare (2008), which is devoted to NR for people with dementia.

It is worth stressing, yet again, that all rehabilitation should focus on what is meaningful for the client or patient. The targets chosen by the people in the NeuroPage studies and by the patients with Alzheimer's disease were goals that were meaningful and functionally relevant for them. Therapists should not decide on goals that they themselves might regard as everyday life items (such as buying an airline ticket). Important as such tasks might be for some people, they may not be part of the daily requirements of a person with a brain injury, let alone a top priority for the person and his or her close family members.

CHAPTER 7

Holistic Goal Setting in Neuropsychological Rehabilitation

Introduction

After a brain injury, a patient's life goals may be shattered. NR should assist patients to think about new life goals, what they want to achieve, and the steps they need to take toward reaching their objective. The aim of NR is to improve quality of life, rather than return to a premorbid level of functioning, as is advocated in traditional rehabilitation approaches. Often the experience of suffering a brain injury changes peoples' perspective on life and therefore rehabilitation goals may be about trying or acquiring new skills that enable the person to live life more holistically than before. This may involve goals aimed at changing unhelpful patterns of behavior that have been a long-standing feature of how they lived life premorbidly.

A recent book edited by Siegert and Levack (2017) covers all aspects of goal setting including theory, history, ethics, and goals for different patient groups. This book is well worth reading for anybody involved in goal setting and goal planning. The authors state, "There is general agreement that goal setting is a hallmark of contemporary rehabilitation and that skills in goal setting characterize those health professionals who work in this field" (p. 4). Goals help us to provide direction for rehabilitation, identify priorities for intervention, evaluate progress, and break things down into achievable steps. They also promote team working and ensure better outcomes. Nair and Wade (2003) remind us that better outcomes are achieved when a patient's life goals are incorporated into a management program. Life goals are addressed in the following chapter.

Almost every rehabilitation service uses goal setting to plan rehabilitation (Evans & Krasny-Pacini, 2017). It has been established that rehabilitation should (1) focus on goals relevant to a patient's own everyday life; (2) be implemented in the environment where the patient lives, or, if this is not possible, be generalized to this setting; (3) be collaborative; and (4) aim to reduce disability and improve real-life functioning. Goal setting should be used to plan and, to some extent, evaluate, rehabilitation. Cognitive, emotional, and social goals should be included. The person with a brain injury, family members, and rehabilitation staff should all be involved in the negotiating process. Although there may be times or stages in the recovery process where it is appropriate to focus on impairments, the majority of goals for those engaged in NR should address disabilities that impact on activities and handicaps that limit participation in society (World Health Organization, 2001).

The World Health Organization *International Classification of Functioning, Disability and Health*

In 1980, the WHO wanted to provide a standard language and framework for the description of health and health-related states. It published the *International Classification of Impairments, Disabilities, and Handicaps* (WHO, 1980). "Impairments" referred to a loss or abnormality of function such as paraplegia or memory functioning. "Disabilities" were seen as problems resulting from impairments, so, for example, an inability to walk would be a disability resulting from paraplegia, or being unable to remember to take medication might result from a memory impairment. "Handicaps" were classified as limitations imposed by society; thus, people with severe memory problems may not be handicapped in environments where there are no demands made on their memory. Similarly, if someone reminds or accompanies a memory-impaired person when it is time to go to take medication, go to the toilet, or to eat dinner, he or she might not be considered limited socially.

This classification system was later redefined and changed to the *International Classifications of Functioning, Disability, and Health* (ICF; WHO, 2001). "Body functions and structures" and "activities and participation" became the terms used for measuring the health of individuals and populations, rather than just focusing on impaired functioning. This system was officially endorsed by all 191 WHO member states at the 54th World Health Assembly on May 22, 2001, and became the international standard to describe and measure health and disability. The old "impairments" became the new "loss or abnormality of a body function" or structure, such as arm weakness or poor memory; the old term "disabilities" was replaced by the new term "activities limitation," such as difficulty in the performance of a task like washing oneself or remembering appointments. The old term "handicaps" was replaced by "participation restrictions," such as difficulty participating in previous life roles (e.g., reduced socialization with friends or reduced occupational function).

Rene Stolwyk (personal communication, 2017) gives an example of how this framework can be used to illustrate attention problems following brain injury. The old "impairment" becomes "loss of body function," which could be described as "poor focused attention," "poor divided attention," and/or "reduced speed of processing." These problems lead to "activity limitation" in the sense that the person is now "easily distracted during conversation"; he or she "fatigues quickly on tasks" and is "slow completing tasks." How does this restrict "participation"? Well, the person now has "reduced ability to talk to and engage with friends" and he or she is "less able to engage in hobbies such as reading or watching television."

When we are faced with the myriad problems faced by survivors of brain injury and unsure what to treat, the ICF provides a framework to help guide the process, particularly with regard to holistic goal setting. In the early days following a brain injury, families are concerned with whether or not the patient will survive. At this stage, clinical neuropsychologists support the families in their emotional turmoil. Once survival is no longer a threat, patients and families tend to be more concerned with physical problems (e.g., will he or she ever walk again) or they may, for example, be worried at their relatives' lack of speech, or visual appearance (e.g., secondary to a craniectomy). Our role at this acute stage of recovery is to help reduce loss of body function such as retraining walking or enabling people to talk again. Cognitive, emotional, behavioral, and psychosocial problems may not be an issue until much later, yet it is these problems that in the end are more disabling than the physical ones.

In the words of Khan, Baguley, and Cameron (2003), "Cognitive and behavioral changes, difficulties maintaining personal relationships and coping with school and work are reported by survivors as more disabling than any residual physical deficits" (p. 209). These are the problems with activities and participation; people struggle to interact with others, make decisions, lead independent lives, and so forth. Dealing with activity limitations and participation restrictions is almost certainly where our main involvement lies. Personal, environmental, and social factors also impact a person's functions, activities, and participation. Personal factors include one's attitudes, beliefs, and personality; environmental factors include the community in which one lives and works and how much help is available; Social factors cover one's cultural norms, legal issues, and attitudes toward disability. All these factors should be taken into account when designing any intervention.

What Is a Goal?

What do we mean by a "goal"? Wade (1999) suggests that "a goal is the state or change in state that is hoped or intended for an intervention or course of action to achieve." It identifies a client's anticipated level of functioning at a specified future date. As Evans and Krasny-Pacini (2017) note, goal planning has a long history in business and sport and it has certainly been used in brain injury rehabilitation since at least 1975 (Houts & Scott, 1975).

A goal is something that the patient or client will do and wants to do. It should reflect the patient or client's longer-term targets/aims or steps toward them. Goals should be functional, relevant, and meaningful. Where appropriate, they should reflect interdisciplinary input. Although other people may have a role in helping the client achieve his or her goal, actions that someone other than the client has to do are not goals (Winson et al., 2017).

Principles of Goal Setting

First, patients should be involved in setting and negotiating their own goals. After all, one of the main purposes of rehabilitation is to enable patients to achieve their personal goals. In some cases, such as when the patient is in a minimally conscious state, he or she cannot be involved in negotiating goals, but family members and other staff can certainly be included in discussions. There is an art to negotiating goals. If patients want to regain their lost memory or return to life as it was before, and staff believe this is impossible, we can suggest that we try to help the patient achieve a step on the way to the goal. So, we might say, "Well, maybe that is too big a step for now, but we can help you take your medication independently or remember what you have to do each day. Shall we start with that?" Some questions that might be useful to ask to begin the process are:

"What activities do you want to do that you are not doing at the moment?"
"If you were to focus on one thing for yourself what would it be?"
"What activities do you need help with that you would rather do yourself?"
"What are your concerns about returning to work, home, school, or leisure?"
"Imagine it is the end of the rehabilitation program; what would

you like to be different for you compared to how things are now?"

Second, the goals should be reasonable: we would not expect a patient with a spinal cord injury to walk again or an amnesic patient to regain his or her memory. The goals should describe the patient's behavior; we would not, for example, say "improve concentration" because this is too vague and impossible to measure. We might, instead, say that "Tom should be able to work for 10 minutes at a type-writer in occupational therapy before leaving the desk."

Third, a deadline should be set and, fourth, the approach to be used should be spelled out specifically and clearly enough so that any-one reading it would know what to do. Locke and Latham (2002) sug-gested that specific, challenging goals tend to lead to better outcomes than goals framed in terms of just doing one's best, at least in the business and sports world. Gauggel and Fischer (2001) and Gauggel and Bilino (2002) suggest that this is also true in brain injury reha-bilitation. Studies by Gauggel and colleagues have found evidence that assigning specific, difficult goals to patients with brain injuries of different etiologies leads to a significantly better performance than assigning easy, unspecific goals.

We try to make certain that the goals set for patients are mean-ingful and functionally relevant. When referring to "meaningful functional activity," we are referring to all daily activities that form the basis for social participation. These can be categorized into voca-tional, educational, recreational, social, and independent living activi-ties. It is through participation in these areas that we gain a sense of purpose and meaning in our lives. Although we may not think about this consciously in everyday life, activity enables us to achieve certain aims or ambitions that are personally significant to us and thereby contribute to our sense of identity. The focus of any goal-setting pro-cess should be on the patient's strengths and needs rather than on his or her weaknesses and disabilities. The wording of the goals should be comfortable for patients and should allow them to feel they have ownership of the goal.

Goals Should Be SMART

SMART is an acronym standing for **S**pecific, **M**easurable, **A**chievable, **R**ealistic, and with a **T**ime frame (although there are variations on this scheme; thus, *realistic* may be phrased as *relevant*, and *achievable* may be phrased as *achievable but challenging*: Evans & Krasny-Pacini, 2017). *Specific* implies that the behavior should be spelled out such as "Kate will use her wheelchair to go to the nearby post office alone." *Measuring* the behavior is sometimes easy; one can measure the time it takes, how frequently the behavior occurs, or whether it is achieved within so many minutes or, in Kate's case the number of times she went to the post office alone (this was "never" in the baseline period, as she was too afraid to go alone). Sometimes, however, it is difficult to *measure* the behavior directly. If we are concerned about improving someone's self-confidence, or how intelligible his or her speech is, we have to utilize rating scales or someone's perception of this behavior. Any goal set should be, at least potentially, *achievable* but, as we learned earlier, it should also be challenging. Kate could manage her electrical wheelchair well enough to go to the post office, but was frightened to do so, so it was felt that this goal was *achievable*. The goal should also be *realistic* and meaningful for the person; we would not set a goal that lacked purpose such as touching one's nose or improving a score on a neuropsychological test. The post office goal was meaningful and *realistic* for Kate as part of her long-term aim of being more independent.

The *time frame* is variable. So, for someone in the hospital, the goal might be expected to be achieved within 1 or 2 weeks. For someone in a long-term rehabilitation program, however, the goals might be expected to be achieved by the end of the program. In this case, short-term goals and action plans will probably be set to achieve long-term goals. For someone whose long-term goal is to travel alone by public transportation, the first short-term goal might be to travel one stop on the bus with her psychologist sitting beside her. The second short-term goal would be to travel the same distance with her psychologist sitting in the seat behind her; then the psychologist would sit a few rows behind, then travel behind the bus in his car, and so forth. Each short-term goal would be achieved in 1 or 2 weeks. In fact, these were actual long-term and short-term goals set for Caroline who had been attacked on a train by a man with a hunting knife (Evans & Williams, 2009). Kate's *time frame* was to go to the post office within 2 weeks and this was achieved (Wilson, 2009). There are those, however, who feel SMART goals are too restrictive (McPherson, Kayes, & Kersten, 2017). We return to this concept in the following chapter.

The goals set will differ according to the time elapsed since the injury and the severity of brain damage. Thus, a goal for a patient in the minimally conscious state might be "Look at the person giving attention" or "establish a yes/no response." Goals for a patient in the acute stage might be "maintain eye contact and engage in a conversation for 2 minutes in a quiet room with no distractions." Patients in the early stages may be changing rapidly and the goals may be more short-term, but this is no reason why they should not be patient-oriented and multidisciplinary. Patients with a disorder of consciousness will not be able to negotiate their goals, but their families and staff working closely with the patient can certainly be involved in the negotiation. In the later stage, patients typical of those seen in many of our rehabilitation centers are more likely to have goals that involve driving, return to work, using compensatory systems, and so forth.

An Example of a SMART Memory Goal

An example of a SMART memory goal might be for "Jane to remember to take her medication twice a day without prompts from her caregivers; at the end of 6 weeks she will achieve this result at least 75% of the time." This is specific; it is measurable, as we can count how many times Jane does this before we begin treatment; we believe it is potentially achievable; it is a realistic step in Jane's long-term goal of becoming independent; and we have specified a time frame by which this goal should be achieved. The first short-term goal might be to provide a pager for Jane and see if she can respond to a test message; this might be followed by giving her a checklist to complete when she carries out the test message. Jane's occupational therapist will observe to make sure Jane completes the checklist accurately and so forth. Jane will probably be working on other goals at the same time and these may well be other memory goals, other cognitive goals, emotional goals, leisure goals, and so forth. An example of a social goal (anger management) might be "Bill will reduce his expressions of anger (swearing and shouting) toward others, as rated by himself and his partner and as measured by staff." The first short-term goal might be written as "Bill will attend the anger management group for the next 2 weeks to learn about 'triggers' and relaxation strategies." A mood goal for someone with high anxiety might be "Claire will reduce her feelings of anxiety as rated by herself and her psychologist by the end of the program." The first short-term goal to be achieved at the end of week 1 is that "Claire will listen to the relaxation tape made especially for her each evening and learn relaxation strategies." The second short-term goal is that "Claire will practice these strategies each time she feels anxious."

Plans of Action

Plans of action involve staff and patient activity and are associated with specific short-term goals. For example, if the long-term goal for Joe is for him to use a memory system to remember what he has to do each day, the first short-term goal might be for Joe to select a compensatory memory aid to try out for a week. The *plan of action* might be for Joe's psychologist to take Joe to the memory aids resource center to look at aids and to arrange for Joe to borrow an electronic aid to try out for a week. Plans of action should be clearly documented for each short-term goal. These plans should state what will be done, how this will be achieved, and who will do what. In the example of Kate and the post office described above, the action plans of her parents involved converting their garage into a self-contained flat for Kate to help her achieve her long-term goal of independence.

Goal Attainment Scaling

Goal Attainment Scaling (GAS) is a standardized goal-setting approach that pulls together all the processes described above in a formal procedure. It applies an intraindividual method of measurement to the goals to facilitate comparison between individuals (i.e., like the idiographic approach to personality measurement). In other words, it converts predetermined ordinal-level data into a standardized numerical scale, thereby facilitating interval-level analysis of the resulting data. It was designed to facilitate comparison between services who want to know about the degree of change brought about by a rehabilitation program.

Like SMART, GAS advocates measure achievement of goals via behaviorally defined outcomes (i.e., the goal should specify *who* will achieve *what, how often* and *when*). The difference between SMART and GAS is that SMART goals only behaviorally define the desired outcome, whereas with GAS the potential behavioral outcomes of a goal are predefined as a scale. Within neurorehabilitation services within the United Kingdom, the baseline level is usually set as –1, and the expected level of outcome is 0. GAS also defines what would be taken as representation of an underachievement (–2) and overachievement of the goal (+1, +2) (see Figure 7.1). In addition, GAS formally captures the "short-term goals" and "plans of action" that were described earlier in this chapter as "steps to achieve," which are detailed on the record sheet (see Figure 7.1). In clinical practice, GAS functions like a care plan, which reduces the onerousness of completing outcome measures and clinical notes. Every action taken by the patient or treating team is recorded in the steps to achievement section, thereby providing a complete narrative of the rehabilitation intervention. This can be used therapeutically to support patients to reflect on the rehabilitation process and barriers to change, which can be particularly useful when dealing with people with poor insight, memory problems, or organic personality disorder with a tendency only to be able to focus attention on the immediate moment (i.e., they struggle to reflect on patterns of behavior that are causing them to fail to progress).

Client:	T-score start:		T-score end:	Completed by:
GAS setting date:	Review date:		Client level of involvement:	Signature:

PROBLEM:

Level of predicted outcome	Goal No.	Weight of goal	Subject area	X / ✓	Steps to achievement
MUCH LESS THAN EXPECTED LEVEL OF OUTCOME (−2)					
LESS THAN EXPECTED LEVEL OF OUTCOME (−1)					
EXPECTED LEVEL OF OUTCOME (0)					
BETTER THAN EXPECTED LEVEL OF OUTCOME (1)					
MUCH BETTER THAN EXPECTED LEVEL OF OUTCOME (2)					
VARIANCE CODE					

FIGURE 7.1. Goal Attainment Scaling form (original version). Reprinted with attribution under the terms of the open governance license; Donna Underwood on behalf of the Homerton University Hospital NHS Foundation Trust.

From *Essentials of Neuropsychological Rehabilitation* by Barbara A. Wilson and Shai Betteridge. Copyright © 2019 The Guilford Press. Permission to photocopy this figure is granted to purchasers of this book for personal use or use with individual patients (see copyright page for details). Purchasers can download and print enlarged versions of this figure (see the box at the end of the table of contents).

Another attractive feature of GAS is that the patient is required to rate how important the goal is to him or her on a scale of 1–5, where 1 represents least important and 5 most important. This self-assessment of the patient's motivational level is incredibly valuable to the therapeutic process. Often patients can be highly compliant and amenable with health professionals. Consequently, therapists can feel like they have facilitated a collaborative goal-setting process, but in reality the patient was just being a "good patient" rather than expressing his or her true values, beliefs, and aspirations. This results in goals being therapy-led rather than patient-centered. However, in the authors' experience, patients are often very honest about rating the importance of a goal, and this can help the therapist prioritize interventions. Exploring why a goal has a low importance value with the patient can also help elicit barriers to change.

GAS was originally developed for use with mental health patients (Kiresuk & Sherman, 1968) to capture the fluctuations in their presentation, especially the tendency for their condition to deteriorate. Hence, the scaling of the outcomes ranges from –2 to +2. GAS has since been adopted and used by health professionals working with lots of different populations (e.g., those with chronic pain, people with dementia, those with learning disabilities, children, and adolescents) and in more recent years has been used extensively in neurorehabilitation (Mannion, Caporaso, Pulkovski, & Sprott, 2010; Rockwood, Fay, Song, MacKnight, & Gorman, 2006; Tobbel & Burns, 1997; Kleinrahm, Keller, Lutz, Kölch, & Fegert, 2013).

Currently in England, it is a requirement of the NHS that all specialist inpatient neurorehabilitation centers use GAS as an outcome measure (cf. UKROC minimum data set; Turner-Stokes et al., 2012). However, it is noteworthy that GAS was never designed as a posttreatment outcome measure and should not be used to assess the level of an individual's impairment compared to his or her peers. Higher overall scores at discharge do not necessarily equate to better outcomes in the individual's condition; rather, they may reflect poor goal setting by the therapist. The objective of the scoring system in GAS is to facilitate better clinical governance of the goal-setting process (i.e., to provide a systematic approach to maintain and improve the quality of individual goal setting by therapists, and thereby to ensure that patients receive equitable care and treatment).

In effect, the scoring system in GAS detects differences in the degree of "realism" of the expected outcomes set by therapists (Kiresuk, Smith, & Cardillo, 1994). The difference between the baseline score and the obtained score at discharge from rehabilitation is calculated and referred to as the GAS score. The mean GAS score (derived by dividing the sum of all GAS scores by the number of goals) is calculated, then converted to a T-score using a formula that corrects for the weight of the goals (i.e., the patient's importance value). The T-score indicates whether goals are being set too easy or too hard for patients to achieve. For instance, if goal setters are overly optimistic and tend to specify expected levels of outcome that, on average, are too difficult to achieve, GAS T-scores will have a mean less than 50; whereas overly pessimistic goal setters, who have set the expected level of outcome at a level that is too easy to attain, will result in T-scores above 50 (Kiresuk, Smith, & Cardillo, 1994).

GAS also has another inbuilt quality control metric, whereby patients are only expected to achieve 75% of goals set. It is recommended that individuals set no more than eight goals at any one time. This is based on the principle that most people in everyday life do not achieve all the objectives they set themselves. For instance, very few of us achieve all the New Year resolutions we set. Nevertheless, having such objectives, 'aiming high' so to speak, often spurs us on and motivates us to achieve lots of unexpected outcomes in life. Often, we may not achieve our original objective because it changes as we achieve steps along the journey toward it. In this way, arguably, GAS mirrors more closely the process by which most of us set and work toward life goals. Playford, Siegert, Levack, and Freeman (2009), concluded following a conference designed to obtain consensus regarding goal setting in neurorehabilitation, that goals do not need to be achievable but should reflect the patient's ambitions, and that capturing this aspirational information is an important part of motivating patients and maintaining patient-centered care.

The benefit of GAS over other goal-setting approaches is that it captures the aspiration information in a formal way. The ultimate objective, or, in GAS terminology, "the much better than expected level of outcome" (i.e., +2 level), is the patient's aspiration, and is not the objective of intervention. Enabling this aspiration to be recorded and openly discussed with the patient helps maintain his or her motivation to work on the "expected level" of outcome from the goal. In the authors' experience, survivors of brain injury often struggle to hold in mind the purpose of rehabilitation interventions, but do retain their aspirational wishes; so, having formal paperwork that details how the intervention is a step toward achieving the person's aspiration is a helpful aid to maintain engagement in rehabilitation. When a patient's motivation fluctuates or wanes, reviewing the GAS paperwork, and reminding him or her how the goal is linked to his or her ultimate objective, helps refocus his or her attention on the goal, thus enabling reengagement with the intervention plan.

Subtle changes have been proposed to the original GAS process to adapt it for use in different neurorehabilitation settings. Consequently, no service is actually using exactly the same approach, which is problematic for the NHS's national evaluation project—although many of the adaptations have been informed by patient feedback and are potentially beneficial in clinical practice. For example, a service user's audit conducted in 2003 at the Wolfson Neurorehabilitation Centre, St. George's University Hospital, London, found that patients considered the scaling of the goal as it was laid out on the page "confusing" because it placed –2 at the top and +2 at the bottom (see Figure 7.1). Patients reported that they would prefer the scale to go upwards (i.e., –2 at the bottom and+2 at the top), as they felt this better represented improvement. They reported that having the scale going downward felt counterintuitive to them. The GAS goal sheet used with patients was redesigned to reflect the service users feedback (see Figure 7.2) and this is the version of GAS that the Wolfson Centre continues to use today and many other rehabilitation services in England have employed.

Similarly, Turner-Stokes (2012) adapted the original GAS process

FIGURE 7.2. Goal Attainment Scaling form (Wolfson Neurorehabilitation Services version). Reprinted with permission from St. George's University Hospital NHS Foundation Trust.

From *Essentials of Neuropsychological Rehabilitation* by Barbara A. Wilson and Shai Betteridge. Copyright © 2019 The Guilford Press. Permission to photocopy this figure is granted to purchasers of this book for personal use or use with individual patients (see copyright page for details). Purchasers can download and print enlarged versions of this figure (see the box at the end of the table of contents).

based on therapists' feedback. This resulted in the creation of the "GAS-light model," which sought to overcome the challenges therapists reported when implementing GAS in a busy hyperacute neurorehabilitation service. The problems therapists identified included:

1. According to the original GAS method, descriptions of achievement should be predefined for each of the five outcome scores (−2, −1, 0, +1, +2) using a follow-up guide. This is very time-consuming, when ultimately only one level will be used.
2. Clinicians are confused by the various different numerical methods reported in the literature.
3. They generally dislike applying negative scores, which may be discouraging to patients and put off by the complex formula (Turner-Stokes, 2012, p. 3).

Turner-Stokes argues that the GAS-light model has been devised to overcome these problems and help clinicians build GAS into their clinical thinking so that GAS is an integral part of the decision-making and review process. The key changes in GAS-light are:

1. The only redefined scoring level is that for the zero score (i.e., a clear description of the intended level of achievement) SMARTly set and fully documented—all other levels are rated retrospectively.
2. The patient and treating team are involved together in both goal setting and goal evaluation.
3. Goal rating is done using a 6-point verbal score in the clinic setting (which is later translated into a numerical score to derive the T-score) (Turner-Stokes, 2012, p. 3).

While GAS-light may be more user-friendly for clinicians and better at capturing the true qualitative outcomes from an individual's rehabilitation program, it also loses the essence of the spirit of GAS. It is no longer measuring the quality of the therapists' ability to predict realistic outcomes from their rehabilitation intervention against a predetermined scale. Defining the scale after the event has the feel of "cooking the books" about it and doesn't fit comfortably with a person-centered approach or the scientific method of evaluation. Nevertheless, it can be a useful model especially in acute settings (e.g., acute stroke rehabilitation wards) where patient turnover is often 6–8 weeks. GAS was designed and validated for use over longer treatment lengths and the investment of time required to complete it is an inefficient use of clinician time in acute rehabilitation where patients often change rapidly and therefore goals are often achieved at speed and therefore new goals need to be written at equivalent speed. Further, there may be limited opportunity to involve the patient in the goal-setting process in such environments (e.g., because the patient is in a minimal state of consciousness); therefore GAS-light is a much more appropriate goal-setting approach in these settings, but it is questionable whether the T-score formula is still meaningful or valid. If the T-score is deemed invalid, then GAS-light is really just a more formulaic method of implementing SMART goals.

Review of Goals

How often goals are reviewed will depend on the timescales for goal achievement but a regular review is essential. It should be noted whether each goal is achieved, partially achieved, or not achieved. If the goals are not achieved or only partially achieved, staff need to document why this is so. Should the goals be reset or rewritten? Should another treatment approach be used? Is there another reason for the failure? Liaison with the rest of the team is essential; there may be a common theme for the nonachievement of goals.

Variance codes may be useful for accounting for failures. These variance codes state whether the failure is to do with (1) the patient or caregiver, (2) the staff team, (3) internal administration, or (4) external administration. Problems with the patient or caregiver include such factors as the patient being unwell, not adhering to the goal, or having difficulty applying the strategy; or the goal being reprioritized; or the caregiver being unavailable. Failures due to the staff team include staff being unavailable, an inappropriate timescale, insufficient available therapy time, or an incomplete assessment. Internal administration failures include equipment being unavailable or a staff post being vacant or transport not arriving. External administration failures include work trial cancellation or unavailability of accommodation or the appointment was cancelled.

Goal setting is the focus of current rehabilitation. Irrespective of the goal-setting approach adopted, goals should be specific and difficult (but realistically achievable). There should be a long-term goal and a series of short-term goals. There is a need to ensure that the rationale for choosing a particular goal is clear to the patient and remembered by the patient (written or recorded information may be required). Opportunities for success should be provided in order to increase self-efficacy. Regular feedback on progress should be provided to the patient and all others concerned.

CHAPTER 8

Using Goals to Guide Neuropsychological Rehabilitation

Introduction

Wade (2017), referring to the skills needed by those working in rehabilitation, stressed the theme that "setting goals for patients is the central skill and process; without this skill, a clinician cannot deliver effective rehabilitation" (p. vii). If the essence of rehabilitation is to help people achieve personally meaningful and relevant goals, then such goals need to be discussed and negotiated between all parties involved. The focus of treatment is on improving aspects of everyday life and, as Ylvisaker and Feeney (2000) indicate, "Rehabilitation needs to involve personally meaningful themes, activities, settings and interactions" (p. 13). Goals may be cognitive, emotional, social, vocational, educational, recreational, or to do with independent living. Wilson, Evans, and Keohane (2002) describe the treatment of a man with both a stroke and a head injury. One of this man's goals was to fly his model helicopter again, an important goal for him to obtain his premorbid quality of life, which would never have been considered 40 years ago. Clare (2000) describes how people with dementia select their own targets for treatments. This is a much healthier state of affairs than providing patients with experimental or artificial material to work on. We stated in Chapter 7 that there are challenges to SMART goals. McPherson et al. (2017) address this issue. In particular, they ask if goals need to be achievable, realistic and in a time frame (or as they say, time-bound). They comment that goals need not always be achievable, because demanding goals, even if they are not always reached, can sometimes bring about positive outcomes. Goals do not always need to be realistic as aspirational goals may encourage motivation, and they do not always need to be time-bound as fixation on short-term achievement may reduce the potential for long-term adaptation. McPherson and her colleagues (2017) suggest a new acronym MEANING—to replace SMART. This stands for **M**eaningful overall goals, **E**ngage to establish trust and communication to determine what is meaningful, **A**nchor subgoals, **N**egotiate, **I**ntention–implementation gap, **N**ew goals or view goal setting as a strategy that changes over time, and **G**oals as behavior change. Whether this new acronym and subsequent changes in activity will ever replace SMART remains to be seen; it is certainly longer and more difficult to remember. Perhaps the main point here is that SMART goals may, at times, need to be challenged. Recently, some of our ex-clients at the OZC said they felt their goals should be looser because what they really wanted was to be more confident, to feel safe, and to be more hopeful about their futures. These were the goals they valued and they felt that the SMART goals were too controlling.

Rehabilitation is ultimately concerned with helping people to participate in personally valued activities (self-care, domestic activities, work, education, leisure, family, and social life). These may be considered as life goals. Nair and Wade (2003) interviewed 93 survivors of brain injury to determine their most important goals. Goals identified as extremely important were the following: family came top, with 64 people mentioning this; second was personal care, mentioned by 59 of the 93 participants; a close third, stated by 58 people, was residential arrangements. Their partner was remarked on by 53 people. The other goal areas recognized as extremely important were social contacts (30), financial status (29), leisure (26), religion (22), and work (19). No doubt, different populations would rate these goals differently, so, for example, if a younger population sustaining a TBI had been interviewed, it is likely that more than 19 would have rated work goals as extremely important.

Motivation is likely to be increased through collaborative person-centered goal planning, because everyone involved is working on real-life problems and difficulties with generalization are reduced.

Identifying and Setting Goals

Assuming that by this stage information has been gathered on the patient's pathology, impairments, strengths, and weaknesses (McGrath, 2008), the first step in the goal planning approach is to discuss with the patient, the family, and other team members what it is they want to achieve both in the long term and short term. McGrath (2008) suggests we determine the patient's motivating values, significant life roles and relationships, wishes, beliefs, and expectations from rehabilitation. At the OZC we will have explored these in the initial interview and assessment. Consider next what needs to change in order to achieve these goals. Does the patient have the ability to meet this goal or these goals? We would not expect a blind person to see again or an amnesic patient to remember again. Can he or she work for long enough to achieve a particular goal? Fatigue may be a big factor if, for example, someone wishes to return to a full-time job. Does the goal need to occur more or less frequently? Thus, someone who forgets to take his or her medication 50% of the time may decide the goal is to take medication each time it is required, that is, 100% of the time. On the other hand, if he or she is asking the same question 20 times in a day, the goal may be to reduce this question asking to less than five times a day.

We discussed the art of negotiation in the previous chapter, but we stress here that a delicate discussion will often need to be made between what the family and/or patients want and how to frame that goal. It should also be made clear just how it will be known when a goal has been achieved or, in other words, what criteria will be used to determine success. As we said earlier, this is sometimes easy but in other cases we are more dependent on people's ratings of success. These, in turn, might be influenced by the mood of the person completing the scale or questionnaire, so we need to be cautious about the scores.

Another problem that can sometimes occur is that a person can rate him- or herself as worse because of an improvement in insight. This has been known to occur, for example, on the EBIQ (Teasdale et al., 1997). Our clinical experience suggests that people can rate themselves as having few problems prior to rehabilitation and then as their insight increases, they may rate themselves as having more problems even though things are improving. The other problem that may occur is that the discrepancy between patient and carer ratings on the EBIQ may fluctuate as a result of rehabilitation (Bateman et al., 2009) or people may improve on recognizing difficulties in some domains but not on others (Bate et al., 2009); thus, they may recognize they have memory problems but fail to recognize their behavior is inappropriate.

To return to goal setting: once a goal has been set, intervention can start to address it. After a specified period of time the goal is reviewed. If achieved, a new goal is set, whereas if the goal is not achieved the intervention may need to be altered. It may be a question of allowing further time or modifying the criteria in some way, or it may be that the goal was inappropriate and has to be abandoned.

Generalization of Goals to Real Life

Generalization should be built in to any rehabilitation program. Perhaps the strategy needs to be taught in other contexts or situations. Or it may need to be taught for other problems or be used in the presence of different people. If generalization or transfer occurs spontaneously, that can be seen as a bonus, but for many people transfer to real life will not happen unless it is planned for. Many rehabilitation programs fail because insufficient account is taken of generalization. If we teach someone to use a notebook to remember appointments in the rehabilitation center, the notebook may not be used in other situations; if we can successfully teach someone to relax and reduce anxiety in the psychologist's office, we do not know that the person will complete the relaxation procedure elsewhere; and if we can stop someone asking the same question over and over again in occupational therapy, the repetitions may reoccur once the person goes home. Planning for generalization should be part of every program. The main goal areas at the OZC are goals to do with understanding brain injury, work, leisure activities, driving, memory systems, activities of daily living, mood, study skills, and anger management. However, the nature and severity of the brain injury as well as the time passed since the injury may impact on a patient's ability to generalize goals learned in clinic practice to real-life situations. Those at rehabilitation centers like the OZC may well be focused on driving, work, and using compensatory aids. With patients in the acute stage, the emphasis is more likely to be something along the lines of "Tony will be able to remain seated and attend to the task for 5 minutes in a quiet room with no distractions." Those people in, or just emerging from, a minimally conscious state may well be set goals such as "Track a colored ball for 5 seconds" or "Switch gaze from one person to another." Goals need to be set individually with patients and/or family members to ensure that they are relevant and real to them. Those with impaired awareness may benefit from education and consistent feedback on their performance.

Some ideas for ensuring generalisation are as follows: goals set and practiced in the hospital or clinic setting need to be ones the patients need or want to achieve in real life. Use familiar objects such as the patient's own clothes to dress with and his or her own toiletries to wash, shave, or make up with. Set up the environment to be as close to that seen at home as possible. Generalization can improve through the implementation of even simple things like what side of the bed will the patient need to get in and out of at home; what kind of computer, telephone, or washing machine is he or she familiar with; and what public transportation timetables are used in the patient's own neighborhood. Some patients benefit from having time at home such as a home visit or weekend leave before being discharged to help with generalization. It may be necessary to educate family members and significant others regarding the nature of the patient's difficulties and how best to help him or her. We may need to *teach* generalization, for example, to go with the person to the new environment and teach the strategy there.

Issues Affecting Goal Planning

As mentioned before, the stage of recovery will affect the goals set. Early stage patients are changing rapidly, so the goals set may be more short-term. However, this is no reason why the goals should not be client-oriented and multidisciplinary. The level of insight may affect the negotiation process. Some people believe that good rehabilitation means good insight, but we should remember that even people in a coma can learn simple tasks (Shiel et al., 1993) and so can people with profound learning disabilities (Yule & Carr, 1980). These people certainly do not have good insight, so survivors of brain injury with poor insight can, of course, learn. Nevertheless, it is probably true to say that we have to set less demanding goals for those with poor insight or to set short-term goals that will raise insight (e.g., set up behavioral experiments that test out the patient's beliefs about his or her condition, such as the information-gathering exercise advocated by Sohlberg et al., 1994). We have also addressed the need for sensitive negotiation of goals. One of the most frequent goals of many people with TBI is the desire to return to work, and they often wish to set this as a goal. Return to work depends on many factors both within and outside the control of the patient, family, and rehabilitation staff. Therefore, we do not advocate setting a goal such as "return to work" as the expected level of outcome from a NR program. We are more likely to suggest more achievable tasks: "X will identify the tasks required in order to return to work/return to the previous job." A subsidiary goal here might be "If return to work is not possible, X will have an alternative action plan." If a patient's level of insight increases during the rehabilitation program, it may be necessary to set or renegotiate new goals.

Other issues include the time available to the staff for engagement in goal setting. In the authors' experience, therapists are often not allocated sufficient time to write meaningful goals. It takes time to formulate and write a person-centered goal in behavioral terms that captures a patient's most valued concepts such as "developing confidence." It can take several weeks of one-to-one sessions to develop good-quality collaborative goals with a patient but funding pressures in services often demand that this process is achieved within 2 weeks. This is unrealistic if we are to truly help patients set person-centered SMART or GAS goals that capture these more fluid psychological principles, which, as noted earlier, patients feel we are neglecting. Consequently, therapists are often biased toward suggesting the easier "low-hanging fruit" as goal areas, and this results in the areas patients really value not being set as goals. In essence, the problem is with the time allocated to the process of goal negotiation in the context of service funding pressures rather than the tools we are using (i.e., SMART or GAS). If therapists were given unlimited time to set goals, we suspect patient outcomes would be much better. Although goal setting can feel like a time-consuming task, good goal planning is likely to produce a more coherent NR program for patients.

Another challenge is that it can be difficult to set realistic time scales. In the authors' day patient NR centers, long-term goals are usually set to last the entire program and each short-term goal to last for 1 or sometimes 2 weeks. For those in acute care, however, a goal may need to be achieved much sooner than this, and for those in a minimally conscious state, 1 or 2 weeks may be insufficient to achieve each short-term goal. Similarly, in community settings where contact can be limited, it is unrealistic to maintain the same goal-setting time frames as those in inpatient settings, yet the evidence base for goal setting often leads therapists and commissioners to expect the same time frames.

More research is required examining the mediating effects of the quality metrics of goal setting. This will include research on the timeframes set for achieving a goal, the correlation between goal achievement and patients' self-rated level of involvement in the goal-setting process, and the length of time allocated to goal setting. Clinically, the authors are aware that there are several advantages to goal planning. This simple procedure makes the aims of admission clear, it ensures early consideration of discharge, it is patient-centered, it builds team working, it makes efficient use of staff time, it can reduce duplication of tasks or roles, it enhances links between different forms of work, it incorporates a measure of outcome, it removes artificial distinction between measurement of outcome- and client-centered activity, and it is useful for audit purposes. However, these advantages are only obtained when the goal-planning process is completed in a person-centered and interdisciplinary manner.

Goals and Goal Achievements as Outcome Measures

One of our great challenges in rehabilitation is measuring outcome. Van Heugten (2017c) reminds us that measuring the effectiveness of our intervention or treatment is an essential part of rehabilitation. How we determine this and how we discover what happens to a person as a consequence of rehabilitation is the subject of many debates and discussions. This is in part because of the very great heterogeneity of patients and aims (goals!) of rehabilitation (Hart, 2017). Rehabilitation is concerned with improving function, activity, and participation rather than curing disease states or improving survival. Thus, the target outcomes are more varied and difficult to quantify than in other branches of medicine.

In acute medical care, outcome may be measured by survival versus death. In brain injury rehabilitation, outcome is measured in a number of ways. These include the Glasgow Outcome Scale (Jennett & Bond, 1975), other disability scales such as the Barthel Index (Mahoney & Barthel, 1965) and the Functional Independence Measure (FIM; Keith, Granger, Hamilton, & Sherwin, 1987). Such scales are typically too broad and insensitive for our purposes. Other measures such as return to work or return to independent living may depend in part on a country's or an area's economic situation and provision of services rather than the effectiveness of rehabilitation. Rehabilitation is ultimately concerned with helping people to participate in personally valued activities (self-care, domestic activities, work, education, leisure, family life, and social life). In other words, the purpose of rehabilitation is to enable patients to achieve personal goals. It follows, then, that we should use goal achievement as *one* of our main outcome measures. Patients may be at the "floor" or the "ceiling" on the Barthel Index or the FIM yet may still become more independent, learn to use a memory system, gain a better understanding of their brain injury, and perceive life as meaningful.

As an example of goals used as an outcome measure, Bateman (2005) used goal achievement and questionnaires to help evaluate a rehabilitation service. Of the first 95 patients seen, 75% were male and 76% had sustained a TBI. Of 676 goals set only 50 (7%) had not been achieved; the remainder had been wholly or partially achieved. On two of the other outcome measures, the EBIQ (Teasdale et al., 1997) and the Dysexecutive Questionnaire (DEX; Burgess, Alderman, Evans, Emslie, & Wilson, 1998), there was a significant improvement in scores from the beginning to the end of the program. Goal setting is the focus of current rehabilitation, so goal achievement is one simple way to use outcome measure. Of course, other measures should also be used in conjunction with goal achievement such as rating scales, questionnaires, other standardized procedures, and measures of independence. A full review of outcome is beyond the scope of this book and is covered in more depth by van Heugten (2017c).

Ford (2017) provides an example of goals to do with mood-related changes after brain injury (p. 217). She describes David, a man who was involved in a traffic accident at the age of 52, sustaining a relatively mild TBI. He experienced headaches, fatigue, cognitive problems, and mood disturbance that caused him considerable distress. Longworth (2017) provides a table illustrating the challenges faced by David, the goals and strategies employed, and the context of his rehabilitation. This can be seen in Table 8.1

TABLE 8.1. Dealing with David's Mood-Related Changes

Challenges	Goals and strategies	Context for rehabilitation
Anxiety, anger, nightmares David had always had high standards for himself at work and at home. After his mild TBI, he found himself struggling to manage everyday tasks and became very critical of himself. He developed difficulties with anxiety, low mood, anger, and nightmares, and he found it harder to manage pressure at work. *Low mood, rumination, self-criticism* David frequently berated himself for struggling with previously simple tasks when his injury was relatively mild. *High expectations, sensitivity to even minor errors* David found himself trapped in a vicious cycle: His low mood meant that he struggled to use strategies and made even more minor errors: the increase in errors led to increased self-criticism and withdrawal from participation, further worsening his mood. *Irritability and short temper with his children* David's daughter asked, "When will I get my daddy back?" *Passive suicidality* David reported taking his dog for walks down back streets, in the hope that he would be mugged and killed.	*Goals:* To understand his brain injury and use strategies to manage difficulties across different situations (e.g., at home with his wife and children, and at work). Also, to reduce how often he had nightmares. *Strategies:* • David was offered trauma-focused CBT and CFT. • To reduce his anxiety about the chance of having nightmares, he used a breathing exercise before going to bed and spent time visualizing a safe place. • To reduce his self-criticism, he visualized a compassionate person and imagined what that person would say to him in various situations.	David engaged in a range of activities to support his return to work, all of which incorporated mood management strategies. David researched, planned, and presented a news item at a community meeting. He deliberately chose a contentious topic, as he knew that he would be challenged in meetings at work, and he needed to build confidence in a safe setting. By adopting strategies to reduce anxiety and develop a compassionate approach to himself, he found he could better manage tasks that had previously been difficult after his mild TBI. David used mood management strategies prior to engaging in problem-solving activities to minimize the intrusion of negative thoughts and self-critical ruminations, and to strengthen his ability to direct all of his attention to the problem at hand.

Note. From Ford (2017). Reprinted with permission from The Guilford Press.

Case Study 8.1. Goal Planning

Tom was 18 years old when he sustained a TBI as a result of a severe physical attack by a gang. At the time of the assault he was about to begin an apprenticeship as a mechanic. He was the oldest of three children. His parents had divorced when he was 10 years old. On admission to the hospital Tom scored 8/15 on the Glasgow Coma Scale and was noted to have multiple lacerations to his face, scalp, and arms. He was intubated and ventilated and admitted to intensive care. His injuries included multiple organ injuries for which he was managed conservatively with blood transfusions and IV fluids. He also suffered multiple orthopedic injuries including a fractured pelvis. Early CT scans indicated that there were small subdural hematomas in both frontal lobes.

After 1 week in his local hospital Tom was transferred to a regional hospital for 3 months of acute management, followed by a further 3 months in a rehabilitation unit. Following his discharge home, he was seen as an outpatient by a neuropsychologist and a speech and language therapist. A neuropsychological assessment administered 5 months postinjury indicated impaired verbal comprehension, repetitive speech with word-finding problems, reduced speed of processing information, poor attention and working memory, problems with aspects of visual object and space perception, impairment in all aspects of memory, and executive dysfunctions including poor initiation, problem solving, concept formation, and flexibility of thinking. In addition to these cognitive findings, his neuropsychologist identified emotional concerns including anxiety, negative automatic thoughts, depressive rumination related to the circumstances surrounding his injuries, and long-term adjustment to his brain injury. Consequently, Tom was referred to the OZC.

At 18 months postinjury, Tom was assessed at the OZC to determine his rehabilitation needs. He was seen by several members of the multidisciplinary team. Communication difficulties and low confidence contributed to the pattern of performance on some tests and impacted on the conclusions drawn. Although Tom engaged well with testing, he became distressed when he found things difficult. Fatigue further impacted his performance and cognitive demands exacerbated his fatigue. Communication difficulties meant that repetition and cueing of instructions both verbally and visually were needed to help him understand tasks. The main problems identified were speed of information processing, attention and concentration, memory and learning, and executive functioning. The latter included difficulties with planning, organizing, decision making, and generating solutions or strategies. With regard to language and communication, Tom was impaired on story recall, word fluency, and naming. His reading comprehension was impaired although his word reading was normal. In summary, neuropsychological assessment revealed difficulties with praxis, attention, and memory, with the latter two areas impacting executive functioning. Tom's strengths were good social skills, lack of behavior problems, and high motivation to improve. Assessment of his mood and emotion showed that he had very low confidence and self-esteem and was very self-critical, blaming himself for the assault.

What did Tom and his family want and expect from rehabilitation? At the initial assessment, Tom said he did not have a good understanding of his brain injury and its consequences, nor what kind of impact they had on his everyday life. He wished to make sense of the consequences of the brain injury on his life, he wanted to start his apprenticeship, and he wanted to feel more confident in himself. Tom's family wanted to help him manage the psychological impact of the assault and consequent brain injury, as well as to support him in returning to a more normal life and to gain a better understanding of the consequences of his brain injury.

With support from the team, the following goals were identified:

1. To make sense of the impact of the brain injury on Tom's life.
2. To understand his practical and communication skills post-brain injury and find strategies to support these.
3. To explore whether it was possible to return to his apprenticeship through voluntary work opportunities.
4. To understand his memory problems and find ways to help him remember better.

5. To feel more confident in himself and more relaxed in his mood.
6. To develop his confidence and skills in practical tasks and using public transport.

Tom achieved some of his goals. The way he did this with help from the team will be described in the next chapter.

CHAPTER 9

The Interconnectedness of Cognition, Emotion, and Behavior
The Basis of the Holistic Approach

Introduction

Although cognitive deficits were, perhaps, the major focus of NR for many years, it is now recognized that the emotional and psychosocial consequences of brain injury need to be addressed concurrently within rehabilitation programs. It is now acknowledged that it is not always easy to separate cognitive, emotional, and psychosocial factors from one another. Not only does emotion affect how we think and how we behave, cognitive deficits can be exacerbated by emotional distress and can cause apparent behavior problems. Psychosocial difficulties can also result in increased emotional and behavioral problems, and anxiety can reduce the effectiveness of our intervention programs. To illustrate how problems may be misinterpreted or misunderstood, consider three patients referred to neuropsychology because of extreme fear, typically considered an emotional problem. On the surface, then, they had a similar difficulty but there were very different underlying reasons for their extreme fear. Consequently, different treatment approaches were required. The first patient, Mary, had sustained a left hemisphere stroke and was very afraid of the hydrotherapy pool. She had never learned to swim and had always been afraid of water. This, then, was an emotional problem and was successfully treated with *in vivo* desensitization. She was taught relaxation exercises, a hierarchy of steps was drawn up such as being pushed to the pool in her wheelchair, waiting outside the pool, through to sitting in the lift waiting to be lowered into the pool, and being in the pool itself. When relaxed, Mary was taken through the first step in the hierarchy several times until she felt comfortable. We then progressed to the next step using the same procedure, then the third, and so on. Mary was seen 5 days a week for 2 weeks. Within 2 weeks she was able to use the pool with little fear.

The second patient, Renee, had sustained a right hemisphere stroke and was referred to us because she was very afraid of walking and transferring from her wheelchair to the toilet or the bed. The physiotherapists said she had good balance and no spasticity, and they could not understand why she was so frightened. After talking to her about her fear in order to build up a hierarchy of steps, it became clear that this did not fit the expected pattern. Renee said the fear was worse when someone was talking to her or when there was a dog or cat present (she had several pets at home). It was decided to observe Renee in her therapy sessions to see if we could make sense of her reports. Observations showed the following: first, when on a plastic mat (just a few inches thick) on the floor in the physiotherapy gym, she thought she was going to fall off and hurt herself; second, when trying to walk in the gym, she thought that people several feet away were going to bump into her and knock her over. The long and the short of Renee's fear is that she had lost her perception of depth and distance. This was, in fact, a cognitive problem, not an emotional one. As Renee was about to be discharged home, it was decided to use a compensation approach to help her overcome the problems with judging depth and distance. Renee felt less fear when she was able to hold on to something so the occupational therapists arranged for ropes to be fitted around the walls of her house. If she needed to go outside or cross an open space, she used a shopping cart. Although it might have been possible to improve her depth and distance perception, we were not able to investigate this because of time constraints. The main point we wish to make here, though, is that the apparent "emotional" problem was caused by a cognitive deficit.

The third patient, Paula, was very afraid of physiotherapy itself. Whenever the therapists tried to do exercises she screamed and refused to engage. Paula had sustained a severe TBI nearly 1 year earlier. She had contractures in all four limbs and myositis ossificans (bony deposits) in some of her muscles. This caused her considerable pain. In addition, she had received some previous inappropriate treatment before coming to us. Her fear seemed more like a behavior problem in that she had learned to be afraid of the physiotherapy because of the pain she was in. It was important for Paula to do her exercises in order for her parents to be able to take her out in the family car and to reduce the contractures. A shaping approach was used whereby the length of time exercising was slowly and gradually increased. Paula was asked to try to beat her previous record. Thus, if she had spent 5 seconds the day before working on one particular exercise, she was asked to try to increase this by a few seconds. If she succeeded, she was allowed to spend some time on the one exercise she liked and which did not cause her pain, namely, head balancing. This is called the "Premack principle," whereby one uses something the person likes doing to reinforce something he or she does not like doing (Premack, 1959). This approach was successful.

The Basis of the Holistic Approach

The three cases described above illustrate how there is clearly an interaction between cognitive, emotional, and behavioral functioning as advocated by those who argue for the holistic approach to brain injury rehabilitation. This approach, pioneered by Diller (1976), Ben-Yishay (1978), and Prigatano (1986), is committed to the belief that the cognitive, psychiatric, and functional aspects of brain injury should not be separated from emotions, feelings, and self-esteem. Holistic programs include group and individual therapy in which patients are (1) encouraged to be more aware of their strengths and weaknesses, (2) helped to understand and accept these, (3) given strategies to compensate for cognitive difficulties, and (4) offered vocational guidance and support.

All holistic programs offer both group and individual therapy to increase awareness; promote acceptance and understanding; provide cognitive remediation; develop compensatory skills; and provide vocational counseling. Several studies have looked at comprehensive, holistic rehabilitation and the findings suggest that these programs can improve community integration, functional independence, and productivity. This is true even for patients who are many years postinjury (Cicerone et al., 2011). Cicerone et al. (2008) carried out a randomized controlled trial in which they compared standard with holistic rehabilitation. The standard rehabilitation program consisted primarily of individual, discipline-specific therapies (physical therapy, occupational therapy, and speech therapy) along with 1 hour of individual cognitive rehabilitation. The holistic intervention included individual and group therapies that emphasized metacognitive and emotional regulation for cognitive deficits, emotional difficulties, interpersonal behaviors, and functional skills. Neuropsychological functioning improved in both conditions, but the holistic rehabilitation program produced greater improvements in community functioning and productivity, self-efficacy, and life satisfaction. Most participants (88%) had sustained a moderate or severe TBI and over half were more than 1 year postinjury. Those in the holistic group were more severely disabled and longer postinjury, yet were *twice* as likely to make clinically significant gains in community functioning compared to those receiving conventional rehabilitation. In the later (2011) paper, Cicerone and his colleagues concluded that there is substantial evidence to support interventions for attention, memory, social communication skills, executive function, and for comprehensive-holistic NR after TBI. They recommended that "comprehensive-holistic neuropsychologic rehabilitation is recommended to improve postacute participation and quality of life after moderate or severe TBI" (p. 526).

In 2012, van Heugten, Gregorio, and Wade (2012) completed a meta-analysis of 95 randomized controlled trials published between January 1980 and August 2010. The studies included a total of 4,068 patients. The researchers' conclusion was that there is a large body of evidence to support the efficacy of cognitive rehabilitation.

Case Study 9.1. A Holistic Program

To illustrate a comprehensive holistic program at a British rehabil-itation center, we return to Tom whose goals we illustrated in the previous chapter. Like all patients after the initial assessment and goal-setting negotiations, Tom attended the basic 6-week psychoedu-cation intensive part of the program. This involves attendance at a group each morning for 4 days a week and individual sessions in the afternoon. The first week is an induction week whereby patients are introduced to each other, to the staff, and to the center. They are told about rules, which include respecting one another and not being phys-ically or verbally abusive. The second week concentrates on under-standing brain injury, the third week addresses memory and attention, followed by a week each on executive functions, communication, and mood. Both explanations and exercises are provided for each topic (see Winson et al., 2017, for detailed coverage of each week). By the end of their stay, we expect patients to demonstrate an understanding of their brain injury and the consequences of this injury for everyday life. They should also demonstrate an awareness of their individual strengths and weaknesses resulting from the brain injury. All clients are expected to develop and implement strategies to compensate for the specific consequences of the insult to the brain, be able to monitor their own performance in using these strategies, and carry these over from the center to their own community settings. We help relatives and significant others to assist the person with brain injury to use compensatory strategies and we also expect them to demonstrate an understanding of the relationship between brain injury and its conse-quences for the individual with brain injury and for themselves.

Based on Tom's goals, his rehabilitation program had three major components: first, to understand more about his brain injury and its consequences in terms of language, cognition, and emotion; sec-ond, to develop compensatory strategies for managing the language, cognitive, and emotional consequences of his brain injury; and third, to support Tom in applying these strategies to everyday situations in order to achieve his personal, practical goals. To develop Tom's understanding of the consequences of his injury, he went through the basic education program with the rest of his cohort, in the context of a therapeutic milieu alongside individual psychotherapy and further detailed assessment for rehabilitation.

During the subsequent integration phase, which lasted for 12 weeks, Tom attended the OZC 2 days a week while integrating back into his own community. This phase focused on Tom's personal goals in more depth, developing strategies for his needs. The team met regularly to assure a shared understanding and coherent and informed planning. Given Tom's assessment profile, rehabilitation focused on developing and testing out strategies established in the field of memory rehabilitation (Wilson, 2009) particularly external aids, rehearsal strategies, and basic internal strategies. Tom's potential goal to return to his apprenticeship provided the opportunity for much of this work, as did his goal to become more confident in himself and in his abilities with practical tasks and with using public transport. Therefore, the interdisciplinary team worked across all domains and goals areas with Tom. Not surprisingly, the speed of processing, attention, and memory difficulties experienced by Tom affected his study skills. Given that he struggled to take in new information, external strategies were implemented. These included allowing more time, reducing distractions, taking in "bite-size" chunks, clarifying information, and repeating information.

Tom developed good awareness of these issues and through joint work between his speech and language therapist and his clinical psychologist, they set a goal for him to use a note-taking strategy in the form of a memory notebook for studying. He was introduced to using this notebook in his sessions at the OZC alongside a specified protocol for making notes. This involved making bullet notes at specific time points in a session, with a brief prompt to summarize the session initially after each 10 minutes and then at the end of the session. The purpose was both to encourage Tom's understanding of the information and to use repetition to support memory. Staff monitored the frequency with which Tom requested clarification on any of his notes. We agreed that he would use the book for 3 weeks before we reviewed whether the quality of the notes supported taking in the information and recall. Since the implementation, feedback from staff was positive about Tom's ability to accurately recall the content of the session. Tom felt positive about the strategy; he felt it had helped him to be more reliable and to recall important information. He had also been able to report back details about the day to his father, which he had not been able to do before. Thus, by actively taking notes, Tom was able to recall important information. His method of note taking allowed both sufficient and the right information to be recorded. Finally, this boosted his confidence with regard to the prospect of starting his apprenticeship.

Tom had gained an understanding of his memory difficulties. He felt that once the information was in his memory it stayed there, but getting it in in the first place was hard. He felt more able to manage his memory difficulties with the notebook but wished to expand its use to further areas such as remembering appointments and telephone calls. Consequently, the memory notebook strategy was developed into a more thorough memory and planning system. After detailed discussion of his needs, Tom settled on a black Filofax (a date book) with the required sections. A protocol to remember these sections was introduced using rote rehearsal methods. This included a "to-do" list, a diary section, a positive log of successes section, a contacts section, and a "how to fix things" list section. His Filofax was used for lists, recording things he had to do, and making notes on practical tasks.

In order to address Tom's main concern as to whether he wanted to or could complete an apprenticeship, his manager helped arrange a 1-day trial attendance at his previous course. This provided Tom with an opportunity to try out the study and cognitive strategies he had developed during the program. Tom subsequently reflected that he thought the study day had been good. He had enjoyed being back in the college environment. He said he had two sessions where he was given a task to do. In one session, the supervisor remained with him and in the second session he was left to work alone. He had felt it difficult to work with the supervisor observing and he had probably underperformed. In contrast, when left to do the task alone, he felt he had performed better because he was more relaxed. A week after this initial feedback, Tom said he did not want to resume his apprenticeship, as he was unsure of what he wanted to do. Nevertheless, the work carried out as part of his rehabilitation program, suggested that, with consistent implementation of strategies, Tom had a good chance of studying again. He would probably be more successful if he was doing something he enjoyed and that was easier. We recommended that a learning support assistant should be available for Tom, especially in the first few months or until such time that he felt he no longer needed support.

One of the goals identified was to increase Tom's confidence in himself and his abilities, and stop being critical and blaming himself for the assault. A mood questionnaire endorsed his reports of self-criticism. Through individual psychotherapy, a shared understanding of Tom's difficulties with self-criticism and low confidence was developed within the framework of CFT (Gilbert & Irons, 2005). This approach has been applied to people with ABI (Ashworth, Gracey, & Gilbert, 2011). In order to tackle self-criticism and low confidence, Tom was introduced to CMT (Gilbert & Irons, 2005). Given Tom's cognitive profile, psychotherapy was adapted to meet his needs. He was helped to practice CMT strategies twice daily for 2 weeks initially, then audio records of the CMT strategies were recorded on to his iPhone and he set himself alert reminders twice daily to continue this practice. Alongside this aid, Tom was helped to increase his confidence through a number of behavioral experiments and functional work with the occupational therapist (see below). Tom made strong gains during psychotherapy, and reported at the end of the program that he no longer blamed himself for the assault, was less self-critical, more confident, and more compassionate to himself. Questionnaire measures repeated at the end of the program endorsed these improvements.

As mentioned earlier, Tom was keen to increase his confidence in practical tasks and in using public transport. A graded approach was used to build skills and confidence in both these areas throughout the program. Given his difficulties with interpreting written instructions, Tom was helped to trial task achievement in which the information was presented in different ways, including pictorially, step-by-step lists with check boxes, and short, one-line instructions. While pictures did not particularly help, Tom felt that rewriting steps in his own words was a useful technique. He used this method to learn how to change the oil in a car, fix a fuse, and check the wiring for lights. He successfully rewrote steps for these tasks and used them to help his family. His Filofax was used for recording things he had to do and making notes on tasks he needed to accomplish if he were ever to become a mechanic. He also developed his use of mobile phone alerts. In one session, he fixed a fuse while practicing setting and responding to alerts. He felt that a standard alert would not give him enough information to support recall of what he needed to do, and more detailed calendar alerts were preferable. As his confidence developed, support was decreased and he was encouraged to help his father in the home environment.

Tom spent some time during the latter half of the program lodging with friends, so he had not been able to develop the habit of helping out regularly at home. However, we recommended that he should be supported by his local occupational therapy services to build on the skills and confidence he had acquired during this intervention, using the strategy of rewriting steps in his own words, using them in a trial (crossing off steps with a highlighter as they had been completed), and adjusting them if necessary.

Tom lacked confidence in using public transport in unfamiliar areas, as he feared getting lost. He was accompanied on a trip into Cambridge (a 15-minute train ride away), during which he was shown the procedure of finding train times, buying tickets, finding the correct platform, and using landmarks to navigate to a destination at the other end. The Filofax was used to support recall of this information. The following week, Tom repeated the journey with a therapist shadowing. While he reported feeling apprehensive about it, Tom carried out the journey successfully, and felt satisfied with his performance. To develop his confidence further, we recommended that he receive ongoing support from an occupational therapist to carry on making journeys in his local area.

Tom's final challenge was to plan a meal, shop for it, and serve a farewell lunch for the rest of his cohort. This task served as a vehicle for bringing together various areas of work, including use of the Filofax, writing down steps for a task, using public transport, and route finding. Tom coped extremely well with this complex task, and displayed increased confidence compared with the early days of the program. He sought assistance from the therapist on fewer occasions, and independently problem-solved more than once. Tom received good feedback from his fellow clients, and reported feeling proud of himself for this achievement.

To support Tom in identifying possible areas of interest with regard to work/study, a work placement was arranged for him in a local garage helping out where and when needed. He spent 90 minutes twice a week shadowing staff dealing with customers and doing Ministry of Transport inspections to see if cars he tested were roadworthy. Feedback from the placement was extremely positive. Tom was said to fit in well, to be extremely personable, and to interact pleasantly and appropriately with staff and clients. While Tom now feels that he would prefer not to work as a mechanic, he felt that the placement had given him more confidence in his ability to interact with others. He took responsibility for getting to the placement on time, and experienced some memory successes. He also displayed assertiveness on occasion, when he asked if it would be possible to be involved in more tasks. It was recommended that Tom be supported to engage in a more taxing placement, to offer opportunities to be more actively involved in work-related tasks. It could be beneficial for him to experience a range of different roles, whether paid or voluntary, to facilitate a decision about his future vocational plans.

Another element of the program involved the provision of education on understanding brain injury to Tom's family. The family reflected that this information had developed their own understanding of Tom's brain injury as well as helping them to adjust to its consequences.

Tom achieved the goals he set for himself. Performance was monitored throughout and the program was considered to be successful by Tom and his family. We employed models from memory therapy, executive rehabilitation, and psychotherapy to help Tom use his existing skills more efficiently and compensate for his deficits. He is currently helping out a family member with the family business.

We hope that through this case study we have illustrated the principles of holistic rehabilitation, and encouraged a recognition that it is hard to separate the cognitive, emotional, and psychosocial consequences of brain injury and that all should be addressed in rehabilitation, the main purpose of which is to improve functioning in everyday life.

Challenges in Providing Holistic Rehabilitation

There are, of course, challenges in providing holistic rehabilitation. Not only can working as an interdisciplinary team prove problematic, but the need to address cognitive, emotional, and psychosocial difficulties together as part of a rehabilitation program can also be challenging. Even when one is part of an integrated interdisciplinary team, it is not always easy to decide who should do certain tasks. Take memory rehabilitation, for example. Should this be provided by the psychologists, the occupational therapists, or the speech and language therapists? All of them have expertise in this area, so our view here is that any or all of them can provide memory rehabilitation. The same is true of helping people to understand brain injury. At the OZC any of the three disciplines can run the "Understanding Brain Injury Group." It is probably true to say that the psychologists need to be responsible for mood work, because their training, at least the generic training provided in the United Kingdom, means that this will be part of their skill set. Communication work will probably be carried out by the speech and language therapists and the activities of daily living by the occupational therapists simply because they have the right skills. Much of the work involved in rehabilitation, however, is not bound by one's profession; rehabilitation is collaborative and we should not be bound by "roles." We recognize that this is easier to do in the United Kingdom than say in many U.S. rehabilitation centers because the billing and funding issues in the United States do not lend themselves easily to joint work. In most British rehabilitation centers the patient is funded by his or her health insurance provider and the rehabilitation offered is decided by the rehabilitation staff themselves.

Another challenge facing those of us trying to provide holistic rehabilitation is that sometimes we work with inpatients, sometimes with day patients, and sometimes with outpatients, all of which lead to different approaches. The principles, however, remain the same even though adjustments may have to be made. If one is working with outpatients it may be difficult, although not impossible, to run groups. Evans and Wilson (1992) ran a group for outpatients each of whom was seen individually for memory therapy as well as attending a weekly group session that ran for several months. There was no evidence of memory improvement as measured by memory tests given to the group members, although use of compensations increased. The main improvement was in terms of anxiety and depression, both of which decreased as a result of memory group attendance. When it is not possible to run groups much of the psychoeducational work such as understanding brain injury, executive functioning, mood, and communication can be carried out with individuals either in the clinic or in their own homes. The *Brain Injury Rehabilitation Workbook* (Winson et al., 2017) provides advice and exercises for those rehabilitation workers who are not part of a team and may be working alone. Most chapters in the book are structured in the same or almost the same way, namely: (1) a brief introduction, (2) the theoretical background and models, (3) neuroanatomy, (4) common presenting problems, (5) assessment, (6) making the links (with other problems), (7) rehabilitation: the evidence, (8) understanding and exploring the problem with clients, (9) developing strategies, (10) bringing it all together, (11) a case study, and (12) reproducible worksheets.

CHAPTER 10

The Uses of Technology in Neuropsychological Rehabilitation to Improve Daily Functioning and Quality of Life

Introduction

The increasing use of sophisticated technology such as positron emission tomography (PET) and functional magnetic resonance imaging (fMRI) is enhancing our understanding of brain damage. To what extent these technological interventions can improve our rehabilitation programs remains to be seen, but there are some promising areas of development within the field of research, as highlighted below. However, currently it is unclear how such expensive and complicated technology can be integrated into real-world settings. In clinical practice, technologies available on the main street are offering better solutions to help compensate for brain injury survivors' everyday problems, and some of the best and most innovative examples of these are discussed in this chapter.

Imaging Procedures for Patients with a Disorder of Consciousness

One area where imaging procedures may have something to add to rehabilitation is in the assessment of patients with a disorder of consciousness. Paradigms using PET or fMRI are increasingly being recognized as useful additions to the assessment of patients in a vegetative state or a minimally conscious state (Giacino & White, 2005). Imaging may reveal some behaviors we cannot see through observations. Owen et al. (2006), for example, reported the case of a 23-year-old woman, behaviorally meeting the diagnostic criteria for the vegetative state 5 months after a TBI. Although unresponsive to command, this patient was assessed using an fMRI auditory comprehension task that suggested that she was processing language. Not convinced that the patient was aware, they asked the patient to imagine playing tennis and to imagine visiting the rooms in her house. The areas of the brain activated in this patient were indistinguishable from healthy volunteers performing the same tasks. The authors concluded that "these results confirm that, despite fulfilling the clinical criteria for a diagnosis of the vegetative state, this patient retained the ability to understand spoken commands and to respond to them through her brain activity" (p. 1402). Since then, scientists in Cambridge and Belgium have employed the procedure with vegetative and minimally conscious patients who are asked to think of playing tennis for "yes" and to think of walking round the room for "no" (Monti et al., 2010). Of 54 patients assessed in this way, five were able to wilfully modulate their brain activity (p. 1).

This demonstrates that it may be possible to establish a successful method of communication with a small number of patients (i.e., 5/54) with a disorder of consciousness following TBI. However, the process of obtaining a consistent "yes/no" communication method using motor and spatial imagery tasks and then measuring fMRI activity in the supplemental motor area and the parahippocampal gyrus is incredibly labor-intensive and arguably requires a high level of mental flexibility on the part of the patient. It would be interesting to see how many conscious patients with severe cognitive impairment following TBI would be able to perform this task. We suspect that a large proportion would not be able to because of severely impaired focused attention and mental flexibility. Therefore, it raises the question whether patients who are presumed to be vegetative or minimally conscious are functioning at a higher level, but we do not have the technology yet to detect their abilities.

Given the current complex medical and ethical debate about end-of-life care for people with unresponsive wakefulness syndrome (cf. U.K. case law Supreme Court ruling *NHS Trust v. Mr. Y. and Mrs. Y.*; British Medical Association, 2017; Annen, Laureys, & Gosserieset, 2017) and the knowledge that the majority of locked-in syndrome patients report being happy with their present lives (Bruno et al., 2011; Wilson, Allen, Rose, & Kubickova, 2018), it seems likely that such research could contribute significantly to delivery of NR in the future for patients with a disorder of consciousness. It currently would be difficult to implement this neuroimaging approach clinically as a way of establishing a "yes/no" response, but it is a promising start, which hopefully will encourage researchers to develop more accessible imaging technology in the future so that such techniques may help us decide if patients have more cognition than we can observe through behavioral measures. This, in turn, might help us provide more thorough and intense rehabilitation to this complex population, who currently often receive little because their long-term needs do not fit with how rehabilitation services are currently funded (Wilson et al., 2016). It does not seem too futuristic to imagine a time in the near future when fMRI technology might have the potential to form a communication aid for patients with a disorder of consciousness after TBI, similar to the way a Lightwriter[1] can revolutionize the life of a client with acquired aphasia.

Wearable Functional Near-Infrared Spectroscopy in Everyday Environments

The construct of wearable neuroimaging devices that could assist with the assessment and evaluation of clients in everyday life scenarios has

---

[1] A Lightwriter is a switch and keyboard communication device whereby the user types out messages that are then relayed through the speakers by an automated voice. It utilizes AAC (augmentative and alternative communication).

started to look like a reality through the work of Paul Burgess and his team of researchers (Pinti et al., 2018), who have been exploring the utility of wearable functional near-infrared spectroscopy (fNIRS) in people with executive dysfunction. Wearable fNIRS devices monitor changes in brain tissue oxygenation and hemodynamics. When a brain region becomes metabolically active, there is an oversupply of cerebral blood flow to meet the increase in oxygen demand. The hemodynamic response is an indicator of functional brain activity.

The wearable fNIRS device is worn around the forehead. It contains a number of near-infrared lights shining into the brain and optical detectors collect the back-scattered light on to the head. Data can be transmitted wirelessly on to a computer while the wearer mobilizes freely in the community, interacting with people and performing serial multitasking. The potential benefits to our assessment and rehabilitation of people with executive dysfunction is huge. It is widely recognized in the empirical literature that there is often a discrepancy between the way someone with executive dysfunction will behave in a controlled testing environment and in everyday life, with deficits clearly evident in the latter scenario but not necessarily in the former (George & Gilbert, 2018). It is hypothesized that this is due to the added cognitive load on executive functions in naturalist environments (e.g., multiple competing demands on attentional processes causing derailment from intention). The ability to be able to understand what drives this derailment is crucial to successful rehabilitation planning.

Pinti et al. (2015) have used this technology to evaluate the brain activity over the prefrontal cortex (i.e., Broadmann area 10) during a prospective memory task that involved social interaction and interaction with an inanimate objective. Participants (i.e., healthy controls) were required to walk around a busy city main street area and in the social prospective memory condition give a "fist bump" greeting when they saw one of the researchers along their journey. The control condition involved touching parking meters whenever one was passed on the journey. The results revealed that metabolism in the prefrontal cortex (PFC) generally occurred 6–15 seconds before the intended action was initiated, indicating that intention retrieval occurred when the participant spotted/approached the stimuli. In addition, different regions of the prefrontal cortex were activated for social and nonsocial tasks (i.e., both left and right prefrontal cortex activated in social tasks whereas only left prefrontal cortext activated in nonsocial tasks).

It would be interesting to see how clinical populations (e.g., clients with a dysexecutive syndrome) differ from controls; but to date this research has not been performed. Nevertheless, the findings so far have important implications for neurorehabilitation. For instance, tasks such as driving may benefit from fNIRS, as it could help detect the early warning signs of various risk factors (e.g., fatigue and distraction), thus enabling us to prompt clients when to stop, or to refocus in order to improve driving ability (for further information about fNIRS in relation to driving, see Liu et al., 2016). Cognitive rehabilitation could also benefit from fNIRS, as it could help us understand the optimal time to prompt clients during compensatory aid training. For example, it could be used to remind a client to set the alarm to go off on a smartphone reminder that is being used as a prospective memory aid. Pinti et al. (2015) argue that fNIRS may also help us study the effects of neurorehabilitation in activities of daily life. This technology certainly has the potential to help us obtain an objective metric for the measurement of plasticity in real-life tasks, which may help researchers overcome the current barriers to implementing randomized controlled trials in neurorehabilitation settings. It is feasible to imagine that fNIRS could be employed within the context of a multiple-baselines trial, with participants randomly allocated to different rehabilitation approaches. Such research designs would be plausible in real-world settings (e.g., inpatient neurorehabilitation services) and would overcome the current ethical constraints that prohibit randomized controlled trials in these environments.

Despite these promising developments in the field of neuroimaging research, currently in clinical practice neuroimaging tells us little about a person's ability or otherwise to function in the real world. Therefore, imaging does not currently meet the essential criterion of NR, which is to meaningfully address problems that arise in daily living. There are many things that brain imaging *can* assist with in clinical practice: imaging is able to identify specific lesions and areas of impaired functioning, it can tell us what connections are disrupted, determine the severity of brain damage, monitor change in brain functioning over time, help with making decisions (such as surgical judgments), and can predict which people are likely to remain with persistent problems after a TBI. At present, however, neuroimaging cannot provide information that could help in setting goals or provide information on the most suitable compensatory systems, or how to teach the use of these systems. Brain scans do not tell us how to deal with emotional difficulties or which jobs are suitable for specific types of functional difficulties. Costly imaging procedures are of limited assistance in helping us design strategies to alleviate cognitive, emotional, psychosocial, and behavioral deficits caused by an insult to the brain.

Other Technological Aids to Benefit Rehabilitation

While we wait to see if imaging will eventually establish relevant assistance in the field of clinical rehabilitation, it needs to be pointed out that there are other forms of technology that do assist in the assessment and reduction of everyday problems experienced by people with neurological damage. For example, some promising developments from a group of researchers at Cambridge University, United Kingdom, has found that a vagal nerve stimulator has proven to be effective in reducing aggressive behavior (Manning et al., 2016) and they are currently conducting a larger group analysis with brain injury survivors (Gracey, 2018). Vagal nerve stimulators have also been shown to have a positive effect on attention and executive functioning in people with epilepsy (Sun et al., 2017).

One of the major tenets in rehabilitation is the willingness to adapt technology for the benefit of people with cognitive impairments. Computers, for example, may be used as cognitive prosthetics, as compensatory devices, as assessment tools, or as a means for training. There is also some recent evidence to suggest that using compensatory aids may increase neuroplasticity in the brain. Thus, in brain injury survivors, using a compensatory aid might be more akin to using a crutch to help a broken leg heal effectively (cf. Williams, 2010; Raskin, 2011). Given the current expansion in information technology, this is likely to be another area of growth and increasing importance in the next decade.

Currently, in clinical practice, compensatory approaches to cognitive impairment seek to bypass the deficit area and teach the individual how to use certain strategies to solve functional problems (Dewar, Kopelman, Kapur, & Wilson, 2015). Independence may increase for those able to use such compensations, and they might enable individuals to either manage their everyday life or to at least reduce the number or intensity of problems brought on by the presence of an underlying impairment. External aids, not necessarily technological, are the most effective and widely used interventions for the rehabilitation of memory impairments (Sohlberg, 2006; Sohlberg et al., 2007) and can also be used to offset other cognitive impairments such as language disorders, executive problems, calculation deficits, or unilateral neglect. An external aid is a tool or device that "either limits the demands on the person's impaired ability or transforms the task or environment such that it matches the client's abilities" (Sohlberg, 2006, p. 51). Use of at least six compensatory memory aids has been associated with increased independence, as defined by being in paid employment, attending school full time, living alone, or taking a major role in running the household/caring for children (Wilson & Watson, 1996; Evans, Wilson, Needham, & Brentnall, 2003). Many other studies can be found that provide evidence for the effectiveness of compensatory aids. A systematic review of seven studies by Jamieson, Cullan, McGee-Lennon, Brewster, and Evans (2014) showed significant and large effects when people used external memory aids. For a recent update on the use of computer-assisted devices in NR, see O'Neill et al. (2017).

A Very Brief History of Assistive Technology

One of the earliest papers describing the use of an electronic aid for a person with brain damage was Kurlychek (1983), regarded as important because it examined the aid's influence in helping the subject tackle a real-life problem, namely, to check his timetable. In 1986, Glisky et al. taught memory-impaired people computer terminology and one of their participants was able to find employment as a computer operator. Kirsch and his colleagues (Kirsch et al., 1987) designed an interactive task guidance system to assist brain-injured people to perform functional tasks. Since then, there have been numerous papers reporting successful use of technology with brain-injured people. Boake (2003) includes discussion of some of the early computer-based cognitive rehabilitation programs and a paper by Wilson et al. (2001) used a randomized controlled crossover design to demonstrate that it is possible to reduce the everyday problems of neurologically impaired people with memory and/or planning difficulties by using a paging system. Reminders on these systems do not always have to be specific. Based on work by Robertson, Manly, Andrade, Baddeley, and Yiend (1997), Manley, Robertson, Galloway, and Hawkins (1999) and Manly et al. (2004), Fish et al. (2007) found that sending general reminders to "stop, think, organise and plan" led to improvements in a prospective memory task. These content-free reminders work for people whose prospective memory problems are due to executive deficits such as poor planning or divided attention difficulties. For those with severe memory problems, however, a specific reminder would be required.

Virtual Reality Assessments

Another area where technology is likely to play an increasing role in the future is virtual reality (VR). VR can be used to simulate real-life situations and thus be beneficial for both assessment and treatment. Rose et al. (2005) provide a review of the way VR is being used in brain injury rehabilitation; they discuss the use of VR for the assessment and treatment of memory problems, executive deficits, visuospatial difficulties, and unilateral neglect.

"Virtual reality" refers to the use of computer hardware and software to create interactive simulations and environments that allow opportunities to engage in settings resembling and feeling similar to real-world interactions (Kizony, 2011). VR simulates real-world environments and situations that can then be easily adapted to the needs and characteristics of various patient groups in order to train cognitive strategies in many contexts, facilitating their eventual transfer to the real world. The ultimate goal of VR-based intervention is to make it possible for patients to become more able to participate in community life. Users are provided with different types of feedback modalities for their performance. These include visual and audio feedback and, less often, haptic and vestibular feedback (Weiss, Kizony, Feintuch, & Katz, 2006). VR technologies are now used as assessment and treatment tools in rehabilitation in general, and in cognitive rehabilitation in particular (Kizony, 2011; Jansari, Devlin, Agnew, & Akesson, 2014).

Experiential and active learning in a relevant setting encourages and motivates the user. This is particularly important for survivors of brain injury with cognitive deficits and, often, poor motivation. Many different situations have been used in VR assessments including a virtual kitchen to assess cognitive abilities during meal preparation in people with traumatic brain injury (Christiansen, Huddleston, & Ottenbacher, 2001); a virtual mall to look at executive functions (Rand, Basha-Abu Rukan, Weiss, & Katz, 2009); and a library-based task (Renison, Ponsford, Test, Richardson, & Brownfield, 2012) requiring participants to prioritize and complete multiple tasks while managing interruptions and new information, thereby necessitating a shift in their approach. The last study assessed seven types of executive functioning, namely, task analysis, strategy generation and regulation, prospective working memory, interference and dual task management, response inhibition, time-based prospective memory, and event-based prospective memory. It seems likely that VR assessments and treatment approaches will become the norm in neuropsychology and rehabilitation within the next decade.

SenseCam and Its Successors

One of the pieces of technology that we thought had a great future was SenseCam, which has now been replaced by other similar devices (described below). SenseCam was a small camera usually worn around the neck that took pictures automatically and throughout the day if required. It was fitted with a wide-angle (fish-eye) lens that maximized its field of view. This meant that nearly everything in the wearer's view was captured by the camera (Hodges, Berry, & Wood, 2011). Originally designed by Microsoft, SenseCam was then marketed by Vicon Revue, and was replaced by Autographer and then Narrative Clip. SenseCam passively recorded experiences without conscious thought, it allowed full participation in the event being photographed, and was plugged into a standard personal computer, so the images could be viewed either individually or as a jerky "movie." A number of studies looked at the value of SenseCam to improve autobiographical memory (Berry et al., 2007; Hodges et al., 2011; Loveday & Conway, 2011). It was noted that patients' recall of events was typically far better when the SenseCam images had been reviewed compared not only to a baseline condition, but also to the same amount of time spent reviewing events written down in a diary. The camera was used successfully for patients with dementia and encephalitis and other kinds of brain injury.

SenseCam provided security, confidence, and ownership of experiences. Browne et al. (2011) supply information from users of Sense-Cam, one of whom said:

> "I was able to go over situations in the privacy of my own home to review things which I was uncomfortable with. The outside world can be very frightening and fast and I felt afraid and thought I would have difficulty keeping up. I was able to review my visits into the outside world . . . and practise at home and memorise different situations and how I would address this when I was in that situation outside. This built my confidence . . . so I was able to succeed when that situation arose again. Thank you for helping me—it is an amazing piece of equipment which I'm sure would be helpful in many areas."

Families and carers felt positively too, with comments such as "Seeing the images brings memories flooding back"; "She is more relaxed socially and less anxious"; and "Sharing experiences again was a sheer pleasure" (Browne et al., 2011).

In addition to memory, SenseCam had many other potential applications: it was used (1) to identify triggers that lead to anger outbursts; (2) with patients receiving CBT to help them remember positive events; (3) with people with autism and learning difficulties; (4) in exercise and weight reduction programs; and (5) in emergency and disaster situations, to mention a few (Loveday & Conway, 2011).

No longer available on the open market at the time of writing (early 2018), it is possible to find Narrative Clip on Amazon. There are also other alternative devices: for example, GoPro and Google Glass. Smartphones could potentially be adapted to do the same or a similar job to SenseCam. GoPro, Inc. (marketed as GoPro and sometimes stylized as GoPRO) is an American technology company founded in 2002 by Nick Woodman. It manufactures eponymous action cameras and develops its own mobile apps and video-editing software. Founded as Woodman Labs, Inc., the company eventually focused on the connected sports genre, developing its line of action cameras and, later, video-editing software. It also developed a quadcopter drone, *Karma*, released in October 2016 (see *http://gopro.com*).

A Techradar review of Google Glass (Swider, 2017) stated that

> Google created the most sought-after sci-fi-looking gadget that everyone wanted to wear at least once. Its hands-free picture-taking and head-tracking navigation were visions of our future, and Google Now alerts were put to good use here. But its everyday uses were limited, and privacy remained a concern. Not everyone got their money's worth from this one-of-a-kind, discontinued novelty.

The advantages include (1) it has a slick, comfortable design, (2) it can easily take hands-free photos, (3) Google Now rocks, (4) head-tracking navigation is surreal, and (5) it is a conversation starter. The disadvantages are (1) it is outrageously expensive, (2) the battery life is very poor, (3) photo taking requires good lighting, and (4) there are a limited number of apps. Smartphones are mobile phones that are similar to a minicomputer; they offer a variety of features that allow advanced computing capability and connectivity including the ability to photograph and video events. One app for smartphones is SnapCam that can be worn and stores photos and videos straight to a phone. We feel sad that the original Sensecam with its features well suited to survivors of brain injury is no longer available, but this website lists the best alternative wearable cameras: *www.bestproducts.com/ tech/gadgets/g3110/best-wearable-video-cameras*.

Other Technologies to Help Survivors of Brain Injury Cope with Everyday Life

We have already mentioned NeuroPage in Chapter 6. It received the first randomized controlled trial of an external memory aid. The second randomized controlled trial was carried out by McDonald et al. (2011) evaluating Google Calendar, which was also better than a standard diary. Many other devices exist including voice recorders, the Television Assisted Prompting (TAP) device, mobile phones, smartphones, and so forth. There is also plenty of evidence for the effectiveness of these devices (Wilson, 2009; Dewar et al., 2015; O'Neill et al., 2017).

Of course, memory is not the only function where technological compensations are useful, and we mentioned some others above. Wilson, Mole, and Manly (2017) describe some new technologies that can be harnessed to help people with perceptual problems; for example, barcode stickers placed on objects of importance can be readily converted into information that may be more easily processed (such as a spoken label). There are already smartphone apps (e.g., TapTapSee, Looktel), which can provide a verbal label of a photographed object. People with prosopagnosia may not be able to recognize others but their phones may be able to identify the unique digital signature of a friend's phone and cue the name. Evans and colleagues (Jamieson et al., 2018) have developed an organization app called ApplTree to aid people with prospective memory impairments. The app is designed to overcome the weaknesses with the off-the-shelf organizational apps, for example, the interface has simple information on the screen and it walks the user through the process of setting a reminder step by step. The data entry is more accurate than with Google Calendar, and unsolicited prompts increase reminder setting. A large feasibility randomized controlled trial is currently underway to evaluate the app but initial trials look promising.

Moyle (2017) discusses the use of robots, particularly for people with dementia, and observes how these can be used to help care for them and reduce their feelings of social isolation. McGoldrick and Evans (2018) are also in the process of evaluating an app designed to assist carergiverss of people with dementia (see *mindmate-app.com*). O'Neill et al. (2017) consider several areas where assistive technology can be used not only for cognitive deficits but for difficulties with time perception and recognition of objects, actions, emotions, and faces. They recognize that there is an explosion in such technology and that anything currently described here may soon be out of date, but their chapter ends with cautious optimism that just as technology has changed society over the past decades, it can also change the face of rehabilitation.

CHAPTER 11

Six Fundamental Components of Neuropsychological Rehabilitation

Introduction

As mentioned earlier, all holistic programmes include both group and individual therapy. The aim is to increase awareness, promote acceptance and understanding, provide cognitive remediation, develop compensatory skills, and offer vocational counseling. We have already addressed holistic rehabilitation in some detail, but here we would like to add the following core components that are required to provide a fully comprehensive rehabilitation service: (1) providing a therapeutic milieu; (2) ensuring that there is meaningful functional activity available to those receiving rehabilitation; (3) promoting shared understanding among all involved; (4) applying psychological therapies to help with emotional issues; (5) using compensatory strategies and encouraging development of skills; and (6) working with families.

Provide a Therapeutic Milieu

A free online dictionary defines milieu therapy as "treatment, usually in a psychiatric treatment center, that emphasizes the provision of an environment and activities appropriate to the patient's emotional and interpersonal needs" ("Milieu Therapy," 2003). Wikipedia describes it as "a form of psychotherapy that involves the use of therapeutic communities. Patients join a group of around 30, for between 9 and 18 months. During their stay, patients are encouraged to take responsibility for themselves and the others within the unit, based upon a hierarchy of collective consequences" ("Milieu Therapy," 2018).

In NR, milieu therapy has a slightly different meaning. Derived from Ben-Yishay's (1996) concept, the therapeutic milieu in holistic rehabilitation refers to the organization of the complete environment (physical, organizational, and social) in order to be of maximum support in the process of adjustment and increased social participation. The milieu embodies a strong sense of mutual cooperation and trust, which underpins the working alliance between those attending the program and the clinicians employed there. In his 1996 paper entitled "Evolution of the Therapeutic Milieu Concept," Ben-Yishay points out that people attending the program are not "patients." Instead they are citizens and members of their families. At the OZC we refer to participants as "clients" rather than "patients." Ben-Yishay suggests that there are two challenges that clients have to face as part of a holistic rehabilitation program: the first is that each individual has to join forces with his or her peers and the staff to form a community to deal with problems in a united manner. The second challenge is that each individual, while striving to overcome his or her own difficulties, will do so by helping and being helped by peers, staff, and family.

We consider that the environment or milieu should be one where people feel safe to tell others about their disabilities and handicaps, safe to express their emotions, and safe to make mistakes. The following definition by Winegardner and Lodge (2014) summarizes our attitude:

> A therapeutic milieu is the creation of an alliance among staff and clients in a group setting in which the clients experience trust and safety through constructive feedback as they develop an understanding of the consequences of their injuries and try out new strategies to compensate for them. Benefits include discovering they are not alone with their difficulties and learning from each other. (p. 14)

At the beginning of the program rules are set by the clients themselves. Rules are sometimes called "guidelines" or another name depending on what the cohort is comfortable with. The clients are asked how they want to behave with each other. As each cohort sets their own rules, these vary from group to group, but they usually include things like "Listen to each other"; "Turn off mobile phones"; "Treat each other with respect"; "Don't interrupt each other"; and "Come to groups on time." Sometimes the clients add rules for the staff to follow as well, such as "Keep to time"; "Give everyone a chance to talk"; and "Make sure everyone is keeping up."

The therapeutic milieu depends very much on people supporting one another, so group work is an integral part of any holistic program. Humans are social animals. We are all members of groups such as family groups, work groups, political groups, sporting groups, and religious groups, to mention but a few. After brain injury, people may experience a loss of role and purpose; they may become very isolated. Haslam et al. (2008) looked at the membership of multiple groups prior to patients sustaining a stroke. They found that maintained membership in a group after stroke predicted well-being. The same is probably true for people with TBI, anoxia, or encephalitis.

Groups can instill hope, show patients that they are not alone, provide information, lead to better behavior, encourage socialization, and promote imitation of appropriate behavior: in short, altruism promotes vicarious learning (Wilson, 2009). Support groups are a valuable resource in treatment because they are important for people in distressing or demanding circumstances. Group acceptance, mutual comparison, and mutual support can be valuable in bringing about change. Some of the former clients from the OZC report that support from their peers was one of the major factors in achieving hope. One patient, Tim (Winegardner & Lodge, 2014), said, "I had fun bonding with the other 'clients' and with the staff, feeling a sense of security in their presence. We knew that if we made mistakes they would be genuinely accepted and this helped us put our guard down. We were not allowed to call ourselves 'stupid' when we tried but failed" (p. 12).

Ensure That Goals Are Meaningful and Functionally Relevant

In 2014 Wilson et al. published *Life after Brain Injury: Survivors' Stories*. In this book 17 survivors with various types of brain injury tell their stories together with the neuropsychologist who treated them. These are just some of the many survivors we have worked with and all, of course, had other goals set for and by them. Seven long- term goals is a typical number to be achieved in an 18-week program. We illustrate here in a little more detail one of the people in the Wilson et al. (2014) book, Mark, who sustained a very serious TBI when he fell 1,000 feet down a mountain in Switzerland. In fact, Mark was one of the most successful clients treated at the center. He improved to such an extent that he was able to return to a high-powered career. His goals were as follows:

1. Develop an awareness of his strengths and weaknesses in a written form.
2. Describe how these would impact his domestic, social, and work situations.
3. Identify whether he can return to former employment (underwriter for an insurance company).
4. Manage his own financial affairs independently.
5. Demonstrate competence in negotiating skills, as rated by a work colleague.
6. Use a computer to record potentially important information for his work.
7. Develop a range of leisure interests.

Mark's employers were closely involved with all of the goals related to work. During the second part of the program, Mark began attending work 1 day a week, shadowing a colleague. This was gradually increased and he was given more and more responsibility until his employers were ready and willing to employ him again in his original post and with no drop in salary.

Promote Shared Understanding

It is important to ensure that there is shared understanding among everyone in the program. This includes understanding between clients, families, and staff. Not only should staff understand one another and their clients and their clients' families, but also clients need to understand their peers, and families need to understand what is happening and what meanings are being communicated. Butler (1998) recognized the importance of formulation (mentioned in Chapter 5). Inherent in formulation is the view that the personal views, experiences, and stories of the client and his or her family are vital to the formulation process. This concept should be applied to all individual clinical work, and should influence the way the rehabilitation experience is organized as a whole. It includes a team philosophy that incorporates shared team vision, explicit values, and goals. Additional characteristics of the principle of shared understanding include assimilation of research and theory; participation in knowledge and experience with other professionals and families; peer audit of the service; and absorption of the views and contributions of past clients.

At the OZC there is a group of former clients who meet regularly. Besides supporting one another, they help with research, comment on projects, sometimes help new clients, and occasionally meet international visitors to describe contents, activities, and attitudes they liked and did not like in the program. Former patients can advise us on a number of things including our interventions. For example, they can explain their experiences and ideas about fatigue. They can give us ideas and provide input on how we can improve ways to manage or assess vision and perceptual difficulties. We have turned to this group when we want help with cognitive training for attention, virtual learning environments, and prosopagnosia. One client, for example, asked about "lack of smell" following brain injury and complained that he could find little information about this issue. He requested information for the common room and this was duly posted.

One of the former clients, Claire, coauthored a book about her story, *Identity Unknown* (Wilson et al., 2015). She mentions the user's group in the book and these are her words:

> The Centre runs a User's Group (a group for ex clients of The Oliver Zangwill Centre) which I voluntarily choose to attend, feeling ready to offer my own time and support for their research programmes as well as the need for feedback and thoughts about changes which may be considered for the Programme. It is also a chance for me to continue to attend and I feel secure just being there again in a place where I am understood, cared about and have a real sense of belonging. It is good to be able to offer support back to the unit. I am occasionally asked to share time with the current clients who have similar problems and value somebody else to talk to in a meaningful way. (pp. 1181–19)

The term "shared understanding" is sometimes incorporated into the goals set for clients. For example, one of the goals set for Tim (mentioned above) was "to develop a shared understanding of the cognitive, communication, mood, and functional consequences of his injury." The following description is taken from Ashworth and Mallyon (2014, pp. 88–89).

> In the first step of this programme, James and his team developed a shared understanding of the cognitive, communication, emotional, and functional consequences of his TBI through Understanding Brain Injury (UBI) groups including Cognitive, Mood, and Communication Groups and individual sessions. For example, common difficulties with psychological adjustment after brain injury were discussed in the group sessions with his peers and those difficulties personal to James were discussed and formulated in one-to-one psychotherapy sessions. This process was repeated for social confidence, cognitive, and communication problems and functional difficulties.
>
> As part of this process, James developed a UBI portfolio. He reviewed his medical records and physiotherapy notes and pieced together the events early after his TBI. He also challenged some unhelpful beliefs he held about certain events, which he may have been informed about incorrectly or recalled incorrectly. In this way he was able to establish a clearer narrative of the events surrounding his TBI and develop a better understanding of what had happened to him in order to adjust to and move on from the injury. By the end of the intensive phase,

James had a clear formulation of the difficulties he was experiencing as a result of the TBI. He demonstrated this through his written portfolio of the consequences of his TBI and description of how these consequences interacted and affected each other.

Apply Psychological Therapies
to Help with Emotional Problems

People with ABI are at increased risk of developing psychological disorders compared to the general population (Ownsworth & Gracey, 2017). We need to use specific psychological theories and models to guide our work with survivors of brain injury. These provide ways for team members to engage clients in positive change and the tackling of specific problems. CBT is one of the most carefully worked out and clinically useful theoretical models of emotion and, as mentioned in Chapter 4, it is one used very frequently by British neuropsychologists. CBT evolved from philosophy, phenomenology, personal construct theory, cognitive psychology, and humanistic psychology (Ownsworth & Gracey, 2017). One common theme in CBT is that people have the capacity to alter their thoughts and behavior in order to enhance their psychological well-being (Beck, 1996).

A wave of new cognitive affective theoretical models was developed in the early 1990s leading to so-called "third-generation" cognitive therapies (Hayes, 2002). A detailed explanation of three of these third-generation therapies—namely, compassion-focused therapy (CFT), acceptance and commitment therapy (ACT), and positive psychotherapy (PPT)—are provided by Ashworth, Evans, and McLeod (2017). These new therapies focus equally on cognitive content and cognitive processes. They also propose that cognitive processing priorities become restructured under different emotional conditions. CFT emphasizes the emotional experience associated with psychological problems (Gilbert, 2009). It draws on social, evolutionary (especially attachment) theory, and neurophysiological approaches to the regulation of distress. It has been adapted for use with survivors of brain injury (Ashworth et al., 2011). Although CFT utilizes many of the techniques in CBT, the focus is on developing emotions of kindness, care, support, encouragement, and validation as part of the experience of these interventions. For example, if a patient identifies negative thoughts and then can generate more evidence-based alternatives, he or she is trained to bring into being feelings of warmth, kindness, understanding, and support for these alternatives. Also integral to the CFT approach is the view that we can be kind, compassionate, and understanding toward ourselves or that we can be critical and even self-loathing. People high in self-criticism can experience a range of mental health difficulties, whereas those who are self-compassionate are far more resilient to these problems (Gilbert, 2010). Ashworth et al. (2017) suggest that CFT may help to refocus emotional responses from self-critical to more positive ones through developing the ability to *engage* sensitively with one's own suffering and learning ways to *alleviate* one's own suffering.

ACT, like CFT, believes that human suffering occurs not because of the content of our thoughts but because of the way we interact with them. Thus, being stuck in unhelpful patterns is not the same as being fundamentally broken and unable to lead a meaningful life (Harris, 2009). We should create opportunities for clients to directly experience behaviors that promote psychological flexibility. This approach may be particularly suitable for survivors of brain injury, given the life changes, cognitive impairments, change in life roles, altered sense of self, and new physical limitations they may well experience. ACT helps people to accept their new circumstances while also committing to their meaningful goals. ACT is not primarily concerned with reducing symptoms but instead with improving psychological flexibility. As Kabat-Zinn (2013) said, it is possible to live a valued life in the presence of symptoms and in the face of adversities and challenges. The converse is also true, that is to say, the elimination of symptoms alone does not also give meaning and purpose to life. Ashworth et al. (2017) point out that there is preliminary, emerging evidence for the success of ACT with survivors of brain injury.

The third of the new wave therapies is PPT, which is the study of positive emotion, positive character, and positive institutions (Seligman, Steen, Park, & Peterson, 2005). Seligman et al. recognize that psychology has a good understanding of mental illness, but little understanding of mental states such as happiness and well-being. Even less is known about how to improve such positive states (Duckworth, Steen, & Seligman, 2005).

PPT is broadly based on principles of positive psychology (Rashid, 2015). All three of these third wave therapies were developed to help people with mental health problems, not those with neurological conditions. Nevertheless, all, including PPT, have been adapted for people with brain injury (Cullen et al., 2016; Evans, 2011).

Ashworth et al. (2017), citing Rashid (2015), state that PPT rests on three assumptions;

> First, psychopathology results when clients' inherent capacities for growth, fulfilment, and well-being are thwarted by psychological and sociocultural factors. Second, PPT considers positive emotions and strengths to be as authentic and as real as symptoms and disorders. Third, effective therapeutic relationships can be formed through the discussion of positive personal characteristics and experiences. (p. 335)

Perhaps the most useful model growing out of PPT and developed by Seligman (2011) is the PERMA model (**P**ositive emotion, **E**ngagement, **R**elationships, **M**eaning, and **A**chievement). Evans (2011) suggested that this model could be used with survivors of brain injury to help us understand how brain injury affects well-being. We recently applied this model to a man with locked-in syndrome, a rare consequence of brain damage whereby patients are fully conscious and cognitively normal but are unable to move or speak due to paralysis of nearly all voluntary muscles except the eyes. Communication is with movement of the eyes. This man, Paul, communicated by blinking his left eye when a particular letter of the alphabet was spoken to him. We wanted to confirm that this man felt he had a good quality of life despite his severe physical disabilities. He endorsed the PERMA model by spelling out that he experienced Positive emotion as he gained pleasure from music, visitors, massages, and so forth. He was Engaged in various activities despite his physical limitations. He had a number of close Relationships, particularly with his wife, other family members, his friends, and certain members of the staff. He felt his life had Meaning—for example, he had recently become a grandfather. He also felt a sense of Achievement, as he was dictating a book through his eye-blink communication (Wilson et al., 2018). For further discussion on psychological therapies, see Section IV in Wilson et al. (2017).

Develop and Train Compensatory Strategies and Teach New Skills

The fifth core component we consider essential in a good rehabilitation service is to manage cognitive impairments through compensatory strategies and retraining lost skills. Compensatory strategies are alternative ways to enable individuals to achieve a desired purpose when an underlying function of the brain is not operating effectively. Zangwill (1947) was one of the first to discuss, among other things, the principles of reeducation, and refers to three main approaches to rehabilitation: "compensation," "substitution," and "direct retraining." This appears to be the first time anyone categorized rehabilitation in this way. In Zangwill's own words, "We wish to know in particular how far the brain injured patient may be expected to compensate for his disabilities and the extent to which the injured human brain is capable of re-education" (Zangwill, 1947, p. 62). This question is as pertinent now in the 21st century as it was during World War II. By compensation Zangwill meant a "reorganization of psychological function so as to minimize or circumvent a particular disability" (Zangwill, 1947, p. 63). He believed that compensation for the most part took place spontaneously, without explicit intention by the patient, although in some cases it could occur by the patient's own efforts or as a result of instruction and guidance from the psychologist/therapist.

The examples of compensation offered by Zangwill include giving a person with aphasia a slate to write on or teaching someone with a right hemiplegia to write with his or her left hand.

Compensatory approaches to the management of cognitive deficits are the most effective for most cognitive impairments (Wilson, 2009; Wilson, Winegardner, van Heugten, & Ownsworth, 2017). These approaches can take several forms including cognitive compensations such as using an intact verbal memory to compensate for a poor visual memory. An example here might be to verbalize visual spatial information by saying "Look for the house with the yellow gate and turn at the corner immediately after this" rather than "Take the second left." There are ways to improve learning such as errorless learning or spaced retrieval (Winson et al., 2017), which some people see as a compensatory approach. More likely to be considered as compensations are external aids such as using a diary for managing memory problems; following checklists to remember exercise routines; using alarms to increase attention to tasks; and employing cue cards to help keep on track during conversations. In addition, we can modify the physical or the verbal environment in order to reduce cognitive demands. Examples here include labeling doors to help people remember the location of the bathroom or the dining room; avoiding certain questions that lead to anxiety or to the repetition of an irritating comment; working in a quiet, nondistracting room to aid concentration; and holding important meetings when feeling less fatigued. Chapter 10 considers some of these ideas in more detail.

As considered in Chapter 3, to what extent we can restore lost functioning is a debatable issue. This may depend on the cognitive function involved and it may depend on how people interpret the results of training programs (see Chapter 3 above). We might undertake retraining in rehabilitation to try to improve a specific function of the brain or we may want to improve performance on a particular task or activity such as improved time keeping or use of a diary. Retraining also helps to address skills lost through lack of use such as using a computer. Computers can, of course, be used as cognitive prosthetics, as compensatory devices, as assessment tools, or as a means for training. See Chapter 10 for further information on this topic.

Work Closely with Families

The sixth and final core component is to work closely with families and caregivers who sometimes report they feel like an "afterthought" in rehabilitation. Lezak (1988) pointed out that brain injury is a family affair. Recent government policies from within the United Kingdom highlight how families and caregivers experience a significant burden following ABI, and provision of support for them is recommended. A number of different kinds of support can be provided—for example, giving information, providing opportunities for peer support, involving family and caregivers in rehabilitation, and offering individual family consultation or therapy.

Klonoff, Stang, and Perumparaichallai (2017) list many of the models for family-based support after brain injury that can be found before describing the system used in their rehabilitation service in the United States, where participation by family members is mandatory. All of the following types of meetings are held: with a family member alone, with couples, jointly with family members and clients, to offer observations of therapies, and finally attendance at a weekly relatives' group. The many considerations that need to be taken into account are addressed in Klonoff et al.'s chapter, including social and cultural issues and ensuring that the family member knows he or she is not the patient but is part of the support system.

Prince (2017) discusses working with families from a British perspective. She points out that close friends should be included under the term "family members." She goes on to say that families of people who have sustained a brain injury point out that being understood is what they value most from clinicians. Like Klonoff et al. (2017), family days are part of the service at the OZC and for some years these have been led by Prince herself. She runs these days for adults and also for children who have a brain-injured parent. There are two types of days: one for older children and one for the younger ones. The purpose of the family day for adults is to help them make sense of what has happened and to understand how the injury results in the observed consequences. For the children whose parent has sustained a brain injury, the format is a little different. There is some simple anatomy using perhaps a brain made of geletine, some games to illustrate cognitive problems, and dance routines to illustrate some motor problems (Prince, 2017). The inclusion of family members is an essential part of any good rehabilitation service and is appreciated by them when they recognize they are accepted as a part of the client's team.

Some Views of Former Patients

We conclude this chapter with some reflections from four former clients who had finished their rehabilitation program and were invited back to talk about their experiences to two visitors from the Netherlands, Caroline van Heugten and Rudolph Ponds (Fish, Prince, & Winegardner, 2018). Before using their words to talk about the rehabilitation they received, there are some points made by Fish et al. (2018) we wish to endorse. The cognitive, emotional, and physical consequences of brain injury are long lasting. Longitudinal data show that recovery trajectories are not stable; rather, both deterioration and improvement are apparent (Whitnall, McMillan, Murray, & Teasdale, 2006). Psychological factors exert a stronger influence on recovery trajectories than indices such as injury severity (McMillan, Teasdale, & Stewart, 2012) and we need intermittent lifelong intervention (Olver, Ponsford, & Curran, 1996). For these reasons, we need rehabilitation for people when they are ready to receive it and act upon it. Rehabilitation may start in intensive care but it is a life-long requirement and should be adjusted as people progress so they can receive the appropriate rehabilitation as and when they need it.

The people involved include clients/patients, families, rehabilitation staff, funds providers, and society at large. There are many potential outcomes that could be assessed. Improvement on test scores is not an outcome most people want. They may want to know that rehabilitation is cost-effective; they may be concerned with measures considered important in society such as return to work, relationship stability, level of health and care needs; measures of mood such as depression and anxiety may be important; goal achievement or other goal-focused outcome measures will be of interest to patients; and so too might be factors that transcend the various categories such as confidence and self-efficacy. What are the ingredients in holistic NR that help with these outcomes?

Four former patients attended the focus group—two women and two men between 23 and 30 years old—all of whom had sustained a TBI. They had completed their rehabilitation program between 13 and 39 months earlier. They were asked the following questions:

> "What have been the biggest challenges for you due to your brain injury?"
> "What changes have your family members noticed?"
> "What were the most positive outcomes for you?"
> "What changes have you noticed since your rehabilitation at the OZC?"
> "Was there anything that happened that left you disappointed?"
> "Was there a point when you felt you were back in control of your life? If so, when was that and why do you think that happened?"
> "Is there anything that you would say is the active ingredient in your rehabilitation?"

The session was video-recorded, transcribed, and checked before being analyzed using Braun and Clarke's (2006) guide to thematic analysis. The data were independently coded and initial themes identified, then thematic maps created and reviewed. The thematic map can be seen in Figure 11.1

Some of the responses cited by Fish et al. (2018) include "The main positive outcome was just accepting the injury and feeling

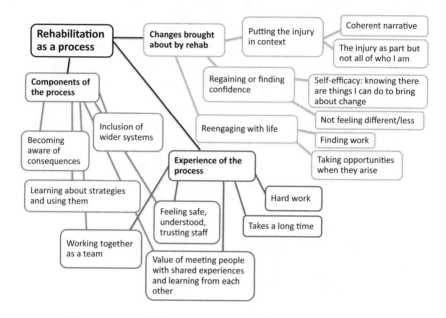

FIGURE 11.1. Thematic map from discussion with focus group. From Fish, Prince, and Winegardner, 2018. Reprinted with permission from the Oliver Zangwell Centre for Neuropsychological Rehabilitation.

confident"; "There were always hurdles to jump over; now it's like 'this is perfectly do-able'"; "My whole life works around strategies now; it doesn't work on anything else"; and "That turning point is when . . . you're not thinking about your brain injury . . . it just rolls."

These views tied in with the core components as can be seen in Figure 11.2.

Fish et al. (2018) recognize that because they were working with a small, homogeneous group of clients, well-known to the facilitators who were all committed to holistic NR, they need to make further plans to collaborate with Dutch colleagues to undertake a larger, more rigorous study.

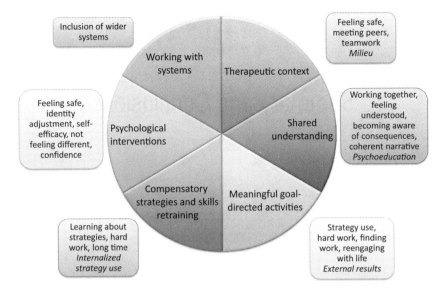

FIGURE 11.2. Matching the core components to client themes. From Fish, Prince, and Winegardner, 2018. Reprinted with permission from the Oliver Zangwell Centre for Neuropsychological Rehabilitation.

CHAPTER 12

Summary and Conclusions

Introduction

In this chapter we provide a brief summary of all the chapters in the book. We have outlined our view of rehabilitation for people with nonprogressive brain damage. We consider how it should be implemented; whom it is for; how people should be assessed; how to set goals; how to ensure cognitive, emotional, and behavioral aspects are intertwined; and how to evaluate. We provide some assessment tools and case studies to illustrate our points.

Chapter 1

We began this book by defining NR and emphasizing that it is a partnership between survivors of brain injury, their families, and health care staff. It is person-centered, focusing on health, well-being, and social functioning. Principally, the process of NR should have meaning for clients: they should be helped to understand what they are experiencing and, if possible, why, and with what purpose. Later we provide evidence to show that NR can be both clinically and cost-effective when conducted as a committed, comprehensive, and coherent alliance between patient, family, health service staff, and possibly other interested parties such as employers, teachers, and social workers.

Our definition is followed by a brief history of NR, beginning with a recognition that modern brain injury rehabilitation began in World War I when the main protagonist was Kurt Goldstein, a German neurologist and psychiatrist whose legacy persists today. Another German, Walther Poppelreuter, wrote the first book on brain injury rehabilitation, published in 1917 and translated into English in 1990. Both practitioners recognized that rehabilitation is concerned with helping individuals improve in everyday life. Another leap forward came in World War II, when the greatest contribution to development of the discipline was made by Alexandr Romanov Luria from what was then the Soviet Union. He contended that psychological research should be for the benefit of humankind and maintained that we should always regard the individual patient within his or her social context. Yet another war, that of Yom Kippur in 1973, saw Yehuda Ben-Yishay establish a day treatment program in Israel, which became the forerunner of the holistic rehabilitation programs so much in evidence today, and continuously advanced by notable contributors such as Zangwill, Diller, and Prigatano.

Chapter 1 concludes with a discussion of issues involved in recovery from brain injury. We consider the meaning of recovery, how far it might be able to occur naturally, and factors such as age, gender, and cognitive reserve, before concluding with an attempt to answer the question "How does recovery occur?" We state our preference for Kolb's definition that recovery typically involves *partial retrieval* of function together with *substitution* of function. Most survivors of TBI undergo some and often considerable recovery, which can be ongoing for years. A similar pattern may be seen following other kinds of nonprogressive injury including stroke, encephalitis, and hypoxia. In these latter cases, however, the organic recovery process may last months rather than years, but psychological adaptation to disability and therefore ongoing improvement in quality of life may take years. It is not true that younger people do better after a brain injury. Age is simply one factor in the recovery process that has to be considered alongside other, perhaps more important, factors such as whether a lesion is focal or diffuse, the severity of the insult, and the time since acquisition of the function under consideration.

The question of gender and whether females are more protected against the effects of brain injury than males is not proven one way or the other, as evidence remains conflicting. There would appear to be more indication in favor of the principle of cognitive reserve. Finally, as to the question of how recovery occurs, we contemplate the evidence for regeneration, diaschisis, and plasticity and conclude that while all of these may play a part, recovery probably involves different biological processes including plasticity of the central nervous system and that behavioral adaptation also influences adjustment and recovery.

Chapter 2

In Chapter 2 we consider who can benefit from this book and include neuropsychologists, clinical psychologists, occupational therapists, physiotherapists, social workers, nurses, doctors of rehabilitation medicine, and speech and language pathologists, all of whom specialize in working with ABI, TBI, stroke, encephalitis, hypoxic brain damage, and other kinds of nonprogressive brain injury. We all work with people who have similar problems and are more concerned with assessing and managing the everyday problems faced by these people than we are with their diagnosis. Others who may benefit from reading this book are patients, family members, general medical practitioners, and purchasers of health care. Following summaries of the main characteristics of the four patient groups, TBI, stroke, encephalitis, and hypoxia, we conclude with a brief description of the main difficulties shared by all groups.

The problems faced by all people with nonprogressive brain injury are similar whatever the cause of their brain injury. Most will have both cognitive and neuropsychological problems. A typical person seen for neuropsychological rehabilitation will have several cognitive problems such as poor attention, memory loss, planning and organizational difficulties, together with some emotional problems such as anxiety, depression, or possibly posttraumatic stress disorder. He or she may display behavior problems such as poor self-control or anger outbursts; there may be some subtle motor or vestibular difficulties leading to reduced stamina, unsteady gait, and/or problems with balance; there may well be problems connected with social skills and relationships; and there will probably be issues connected with the continuation of work or education. Moreover, family members probably do not understand what has happened to the person they once felt they knew and understood. These are the difficulties clinicians have to deal with in NR and we have attempted to address them in the latter chapters of this book.

Chapter 3

The main focus in Chapter 3 is the purpose and process of NR itself. We reiterate that rehabilitation should enable people with disabilities to achieve their optimum level of well-being, to reduce the impact of difficulties experienced in everyday life, and to help them return to their own or most appropriate environments. The starting point is always the person with the brain injury and his or her family. We should find out what his or her needs are, what he or she wants to achieve, and what is preventing him or her from coping with the demands of everyday life. Most of the goals we set will address disabilities that impact activities and environmental restrictions that limit participation in society (goals are covered more fully in Chapters 7 and 8). We looked earlier at spontaneous recovery, so in Chapter 3 we are more interested in whether we should try to restore lost functioning, encourage anatomical reorganization, help people use their residual skills more efficiently, find an alternative means to the final goal through compensations (functional adaptation), use environmental modifications to bypass problems, or use a combination of these methods? While each of these approaches is discussed in more detail, in clinical practice we are less likely to use the restoration of function and anatomical reorganization than we are the remaining strategies. Thus, we are more likely to help people employ their residual skills more efficiently, or to help them compensate for difficulties or to adapt or modify the environment. Using residual skills more efficiently is one of the reasons why we can help people learn more efficiently and why mnemonics work. This is because most survivors of brain injury do not lose *all* of their cognitive skills, they simply have impaired or very impaired functioning.

Compensation is one of the main ways to deal with cognitive problems and this topic is picked up again in Chapter 10 on technology. Modifying the environment is particularly useful for those with severe and widespread problems but also works for less severely impaired people too. Thus, someone with severe executive deficits may be able to function in a structured environment, with no distractions, and where there is no need to problem-solve, as the task at hand is clear and unambiguous. Similarly, people with severe memory problems may not be disabled in environments in which few or no demands are made on memory. These methods are not, of course, mutually exclusive so once again in clinical practice we are likely to use a combination of these techniques.

Chapter 4

Because survivors of brain injury are likely to have several cognitive and noncognitive problems, it is highly unlikely that any one theory, model, or framework will address all of these problems. We do not wish to constrain our clinical practice, so NR needs a broad theoretical base. This is the emphasis of Chapter 4. We begin by differentiating between a theory and a model, before looking more closely at some of the models and theories that have influenced NR. Some of the most influential models and theories in NR over the past two decades are those of cognition, emotion, behavior, and learning, all of which are described and discussed. The most influential theories would appear to be those from cognitive neuropsychology, particularly from the fields of language and reading. We believe, however, that models from cognitive neuropsychology tend to tell us *what* to treat and not *how* to treat. Consequently, they are insufficient on their own to guide us through the many intricate processes involved in the rehabilitation process.

When dealing with emotional problems resulting from nonprogressive brain injury, CBT is probably the most influential method. There have been additional models derived from CBT that are now playing a part, and one of them that is widely used in the United Kingdom is the Y-shaped model, which tries to reduce the discrepancy between the old, "preinjury me" and the "postinjury me" to form a "new, acceptable me."

The book continues with a brief history of some theories and models affecting rehabilitation, including models of learning theory, behavioral psychology, and cognition. We conclude that models and theories of cognitive functioning are necessary but not sufficient in NR. The holistic model, very prominent in current rehabilitation, is addressed. Inherent in the holistic model is recognition of the importance of emotion, and we take a closer look at some of the thoughts on this topic. Keith and Lipsey (1993) consider that all interventions may be characterized by specifying three things: the target; the active ingredients, and the mechanism of actions, all of which are measurable. We continue with reporting a survey of psychologists working in brain injury rehabilitation in the United Kingdom and refer to the models and theories most influencing their clinical practice. The conclusion is that we need a number of theoretical bases in order to deal with all the complexities of rehabilitation. In addition, a good theory teaches us to doubt. We need to challenge theories and models in order to improve science. A model allows us to test out the various components, find double dissociations, and prove whether our hypotheses are true or not. In NR, we need to draw on a number of theories, models, and frameworks or else we risk bad clinical practice.

Chapter 5

Chapter 5 recognizes that appropriate assessment and formulation is necessary for accurate rehabilitation. Assessment refers to the collection, organization, and interpretation of information about a person and his or her situation. Different assessments are required to answer different questions. We can see assessment processes as tools in a toolbox: just as special tools are needed for specific purposes, so special measures are needed to answer specific questions. The characteristics of standardized tests are described and we reflect on the kinds of questions these can answer. The process is then repeated for behavioral or functional assessments, which include observations; self-report measures such as questionnaires, rating scales, and checklists; self-monitoring measures; and behavioral interviews.

We compare standardized with behavioral or functional assessments: the former tends to tell us what a person *has* while the latter tends to tell us what a person *does*. In the former, behavior is seen as *a sign* of the disorder, while in the latter it is a *sample* of the behavior in which we have interest. Other differences are mentioned. We argue that both kinds of assessments are necessary when planning rehabilitation, as they provide complementary information.

The importance of formulation is stressed. Formulation involves deriving hypotheses concerning the nature, causes, and factors influencing current problems or a patient's current situation. It considers the multitude of possible influences on an individual's level of functioning and psychological state. Once complete, the formulation should lead to appropriate interventions. The effectiveness of intervention helps test the formulation, and hypotheses can be modified if necessary.

Chapter 6

The premise of Chapter 6 is that rehabilitation is a partnership between patient or client, family members, and health care staff. Gone are the days when the physicians, psychologists, or therapists decided on what the patients would work toward achieving or aim for in rehabilitation. We now negotiate goals with patients and their families. Goals are the focus of Chapters 7 and 8, while in Chapter 6 we discuss partnership more generally. As a team, we share the decision making as to how to proceed toward achievement in rehabilitation. We feel it is essential for people with brain injury, rehabilitation staff, and others to work together on what is important for patients and their families. Rehabilitation is not about sitting someone in front of a computer to do exercises. As we say in Chapter 6, there is no good evidence that such "brain training" works. Instead, rehabilitation is about dealing with real-life problems. We present some group studies and some single-case experimental designs illustrating how such a partnership might work. We describe group studies using NeuroPage, a system for delivering reminders to people with memory and/or language problems. In each case, the person with brain injury chooses what he or she wants and needs to be reminded about. These might include remembering to take medication or to feed the dog or to turn the hot water on. Evaluated in a scientifically rigorous way, there was strong evidence that NeuroPage was effective in helping people become more independent in their everyday tasks. The single-case experimental designs depict studies of people with Alzheimer's disease who, once more, chose for themselves what they want help with. One woman wanted to relearn the names of her grandchildren, another wanted to recognize coins again, both being examples of working on tasks that are meaningful for, and relevant to, the individual. We emphasize again that all rehabilitation should focus on what is important for the client or patient. Rehabilitation staff should not decide on goals that they themselves might regard as relevant for everyday life, but instead they must be led by the needs of the patients themselves and their families.

Chapter 7

This brings us to Chapter 7 where we focus on goals that are *functionally* relevant to the people involved. A goal is something that the patient or client wants to do. It should reflect the longer-term targets/ aims or steps toward these wants or ambitions. Because rehabilitation should help people to achieve their optimum physical, psychological, social, and vocational well-being and reduce problems faced in every-day life, the goals we will have negotiated help us to provide direction, identify priorities for intervention, evaluate progress, and break things down into achievable steps. As far as possible, the person with brain injury, family members, and rehabilitation staff should all be involved in the negotiating process. There are situations, of course, where the patient is unable to be involved in the negotiation process: people who are vegetative or in a minimally conscious state, for example, cannot make their voices heard. Families and staff, however, can be included. Almost every rehabilitation service uses goal setting to plan rehabili-tation and should (1) focus on goals relevant to a patient's own every-day life; (2) be implemented in the environment where the patient lives, or, if this is not possible, be generalized to this setting; (3) be collaborative; and (4) aim to reduce disability and improve real-life functioning. Goal setting should be used to plan and, to some extent, evaluate rehabilitation. Cognitive, emotional, and social goals should be included.

WHO's ICF is described, as this provides a framework to help guide the process of rehabilitation, particularly with regard to goal setting. We distinguish between goal-setting and action plans. Action plans are not goals, but instead tasks that other people have to do in order to help clients achieve their goals.

The main principles of goal planning are addressed: not only should the relevant people be involved, but any goals set should be SMART (Specific, Measurable, Achievable, Realistic, and Time-based). We provide some examples of goal setting and describe Goal Attainment Scaling (GAS), which is a way of scoring the extent to which individual goals are achieved. We then consider how often goals should be reviewed; although reviews will vary depending on the circumstances, a regular review is necessary. It is also important to document the reason(s) why any goal is not achieved. We conclude this chapter by reminding the reader that goals should be specific and difficult (but realistically achievable); there should be a long-term goal and a series of short-term goals; and we should ensure that the rationale for choosing a particular goal is clear to the patient and remembered by him or her. If necessary, written or recorded information can be used.

Chapter 8

A further chapter on goals follows. This time we discuss the use of goals to plan rehabilitation. We address criticisms of SMART goals, with some clients feeling these goals are too restrictive and controlling. Instead, these clients want goals that focus on hope or improving understanding from others. One group of clinicians suggest that instead of SMART goals we use a different acronym, namely, MEANING—Meaningful overall goals, Engage to establish trust and communication to determine what is meaningful, Anchor subgoals, Negotiate, Intention–implementation gap, New goals or view goal setting as a strategy that changes over time, and Goals as behavior change. Whether this new acronym will ever replace SMART remains to be seen. Life goals are then reviewed.

We tackle the question of how to identify and set goals. Motivation, fatigue, and other factors may need to be attended to during this process. Generalization may also be an issue. If a goal is achieved in the rehabilitation center, will it generalize to other places and situations? Ways to help ensure generalization are discussed. The stage of recovery will affect the goals set. Early-stage patients are changing rapidly so the goals set may be more short-term. They can, however, still be client-oriented and multidisciplinary. The level of insight may affect goal setting and the negotiation process. Even though good insight is helpful, we can still set goals for those lacking in insight. We just have to make the goals easier and less demanding.

Whether we should use goal achievement as an outcome measure is considered next. Measuring the effectiveness of our intervention or treatment is an essential part of rehabilitation, but how best to determine this achievement is a topic of much debate, not least because of the very great heterogeneity of patients and the aims of rehabilitation. Rehabilitation is concerned with improving function, activity, and participation rather than curing disease states or improving survival. Thus, the target outcomes are more varied and difficult to quantify than in other branches of medicine. We cannot, for example, use survival versus death. We take into account some of the outcome measures used in brain injury rehabilitation before ending with a case study to illustrate the principles covered.

Chapter 9

Perhaps the most basic characteristic of the holistic approach to NR is that cognition, emotion, and behavior are interlinked. In earlier times, most neuropsychologists focused on cognitive deficits but for some years it has been recognized that emotional, psychosocial, and behavioral difficulties have to be dealt with alongside cognitive problems. It is not always easy to separate out cognitive, emotional, and behavioral problems. Emotional difficulties affect how we think and how we behave; cognitive deficits can be exacerbated by emotional distress and can cause apparent behavior problems. Psychosocial difficulties can also result in increased emotional and behavioral problems, and anxiety can reduce the effectiveness of our intervention programs. There is little doubt that there is interaction between these functions.

The essential distinguishing features of any holistic program are outlined. All offer both group and individual therapy. This is to increase awareness of what has happened to the survivor and how he or she has been affected by the injury or illness. The person is then helped to accept and understand his or her altered self, perhaps by using the Y-shaped model to reduce the discrepancy between the former self and the current self. In addition, cognitive remediation is provided to deal with any cognitive problems and, if necessary, people are helped to develop compensatory skills. Finally, vocational counseling is offered. In the United States this is likely to be supplied by a vocational therapist or job coach, but in the United Kingdom it is more likely to be offered by an occupational therapist or sometimes by a neuropsychologist. Not everyone will be able to return to work, of course, so alternatives to work are frequently considered. This may be volunteering in a charity shop, helping in a garden center, working at a sports center for people with disabilities or, not unusually, helping out in a family business.

We look at the evidence supporting the efficacy of comprehensive holistic programs where Cicerone and his colleagues have done some sterling work. Van Heugten and her colleagues have also contributed valuable work in this area. We conclude the chapter by returning to the case study mentioned in the previous chapter. This time we demonstrate how a holistic program works in clinical practice.

Chapter 10

Technology is increasingly used in rehabilitation, not only for assessing areas of the brain damaged by using sophisticated imaging procedures, but even more importantly for our purposes to help people compensate for everyday life problems. Computers, for example, may be used as cognitive prosthetics, as compensatory devices, as assessment tools, or as a means for training. We can also use technology for assessment of everyday life difficulties. Here virtual reality (VR) is proving to be useful, and Chapter 10 includes some examples of the use of VR for assessment purposes.

Compensations have proved to be particularly useful for cognitive deficits. These seek to bypass the individual's problem area and teach him or her how to use certain strategies to solve functional problems. Examples are given of how these have helped people with memory impairments. Compensations have proved to be useful not only for overcoming memory problems: they can also be used to offset other cognitive impairments such as language disorders, executive problems, calculation deficits, or unilateral neglect.

A very brief history of the use of technology in rehabilitation is presented beginning with what we believe is the earliest paper to use an electronic aid to help a brain-injured man learn to check his timetable (Kurlychek, 1983). The work of Glisky and her colleagues is referred to when they helped people to learn computer terminology and, in one case, were able to obtain paid employment as a computer operator for one of their patients. Content-free cueing is also discussed. Here general reminders sent through a mobile telephone or paging device may improve performance.

We argue the case for SenseCam and its successors. SenseCam is a small camera worn round the neck, which is triggered by heat and movement and records automatically. The camera is plugged into a standard PC or Mac, which downloads the recorded images and allows them to be viewed at speed, like watching a jerky movie. If preferred, the images can be played one at a time. SenseCam has also been used to identify triggers that lead to anger outbursts. It has been utilized in CBT to help patients remember positive events. People with autism and learning difficulties have benefited. It has been used in exercise and weight reduction regimes and in emergency and disaster situations. At one time we thought SenseCam had a great future but, unfortunately it was converted into a more commercially relevant product and consequently it is no longer available in its original format; although the commercially available products do a similar job, in our experience they are less effective, as described in the chapter.

Other technologies to help compensate for the consequences of brain injury are discussed. For example, people with visual perceptual or visual–spatial problems may be helped by barcode stickers placed on objects of importance that can be converted into spoken information and there are apps for smartphones that can provide a verbal label of a photographed object. People with prosopagnosia may not be able to recognize others, but their phones may be able to identify the unique digital signature of a friend's phone and cue the name. Robots are now being used to help people with dementia. O'Neill et al. (2017) consider several areas where assistive technology can be used not only for cognitive deficits but for difficulties with time perception and recognition of objects, actions, emotions, and faces. This is an area where we are likely to see considerable expansion in the next decade. Just as technology has changed society radically over the past 10 or 20 years, it can also change the face of rehabilitation.

Chapter 11

The penultimate chapter looks at the fundamental components required for a comprehensive rehabilitation service. We need to provide a therapeutic milieu; ensure there is meaningful functional activity available to those receiving rehabilitation; promote shared understanding among all involved; apply psychological therapies to help with emotional issues; use compensatory strategies; encourage development of skills; and work closely with families. We expand on each of these issues.

We hope we have persuaded readers of this book that NR for people with ABI is clinically and cost-effective. The medical profession is usually good at saving lives but often does nothing more once a patient leaves the hospital. Survivors of brain injury are likely to be young, particularly if they have sustained a TBI. In most cases, they will have a normal life expectancy and rehabilitation can make a big difference in its quality. We do not expect our clients to recover to their preinjury state, but we do expect each of them to be able to lead a purposeful and reasonably fulfilling existence. In addition to the obvious humanistic value of this outcome, enabling survivors of brain injury to achieve this end helps to reduce the burden on statutory services for those who turn to drugs, alcohol, and crime to cope with their disabilities.

As we mentioned in Chapter 10, "Costly imaging procedures are of limited assistance in helping us design strategies to alleviate cognitive, emotional, psychosocial, or behavioral deficits caused by an insult to the brain." Repeating this, we, as authors of this book and as professionally committed clinicians working in NR, are impelled to comment on some of the frustrations faced by those of us engaged in this field of work, in which our purpose is to improve the daily lives of people with brain injury and their families. Principally, lack of funding often means we cannot carry out our work as efficiently as we would like. We also face situations where what seems to us to be irrelevant and/or expensive approaches, such as neuroimaging, may be favored above the down-to-earth and often time-consuming approaches advocated in this book. How many times do we see in the media findings about brain imaging? Stories about imaging are far more likely to be reported than successful attempts to teach someone a compensatory aid or to reduce stress on families. Imaging has its place, of course, but pictures, however impressive in themselves, do not address the main issues in NR. They do not tell us what is causing most distress to the patient and the family; they do not tell us how to teach the use of a compensatory aid; they cannot advise us on what job might be most suitable for the survivor of brain injury; and they cannot inform us on how to reduce the emotional consequences to the individual patient and his or her family. All of these, however, are essential questions in rehabilitation. It sometimes seems to us that those involved in brain imaging are regarded in the academic press as more important than the day-to-day rehabilitation workers trying to reduce the everyday cognitive, emotional, and behavioral problems that rarely feature as items in the media. It is particularly painful for us when exponents of imaging claim their research is directly related to improving the daily lives of brain-injured people. We ask readers of this book to imagine they have a relative with a severe brain injury and decide whether money should be spent on the imagers or the providers of holistic rehabilitation? Another frustration we face is the rise of "brain training." We know that there is no good evidence that such training works (see Chapter 6) yet funding providers, researchers, and the media continue to be endeared by such approaches. To date, no brain-training intervention has been successful at teaching people to manage problems arising in everyday life. When patients talk about the impact of their brain injury, they describe the roles they have lost in everyday life, and it is these roles they wish to recover, not the neural pathway damaged by the brain injury. Yet there is clearly something satisfying about feeling that you are "repairing the brain" and this human desire to be able to repair oneself, like the desire to thwart aging, seems to be why brain-training approaches remain so attractive to patients. The danger is that in some rehabilitation centers such training is all that is provided by way of cognitive or neuropsychological rehabilitation. We have been to centers claiming to provide NR and been shown a room full of computers with patients sitting in front of a computer screen engaged in cognitive exercises. To the best of our knowledge, there are no long-term follow-up studies exploring patients' psychological well-being and community reintegration after such programs. Again, computers have a place in NR but practicing exercises on a computer is *not* NR as we understand it. The fundamental guiding principle of NR must always be to improve quality of life for patients and their families. They deserve the best, NR cannot be rushed and it may be expensive in the short term, but it is nevertheless cost-effective in the long term. A civilized society should deliver good medical care to all its citizens and this care should include comprehensive NR.

References

Alderman, N., Fry, R. K., & Youngson, H. A. (1995). Improvement of self-monitoring skills, reduction of behaviour disturbance and the dysexecutive syndrome: Comparison of response cost and a new programme of self-monitoring training. *Neuropsychological Rehabilitation, 5,* 193–221.

Allen, R. E., Fowler, H. W., & Fowler, F. G. (1990). *The concise Oxford dictionary of current English.* Oxford, UK: Oxford University Press.

Annen, J., Laureys, S., & Gosseries, O. (2017). People with disorders of consciousness. In B. A. Wilson, J. Winegardner, C. van Heugten, & T. Ownsworth (Eds.), *Neuropsychological rehabilitation: The international handbook* (pp. 298–310). Abingdon, UK: Routledge.

Ashworth, F., Evans, J. J., & McLeod, H. (2017). Third wave cognitive and behavioural therapies: Compassion focused therapy, acceptance and commitment therapy and positive psychotherapy. In B. A. Wilson, J. Winegardner, C. van Heugten, & T. Ownsworth (Eds.), *Neuropsychological rehabilitation: The international handbook* (pp. 327–339). Abingdon, UK: Routledge.

Ashworth, F., Gracey, F., & Gilbert, P. (2011). Compassion focused therapy after traumatic brain injury: Theoretical foundations and a case illustration. *Brain Impairment, 12,* 128–139.

Ashworth, F., & Mallyon, J. (2014). James's story: Returning from the "dark side." In B. A. Wilson, J. Winegardner, & F. Ashworth, *Life after brain injury: Survivors' stories.* Hove, UK: Psychology Press.

Attella, M. J., Nattinville, A., & Stein, D. G. (1987). Hormonal state affects recovery from frontal cortex lesions in adult female rats. *Behavioral and Neural Biology, 48,* 352–367.

Baddeley, A. D. (1993). A theory of rehabilitation without a model of learning is a vehicle without an engine: A comment on Caramazza and Hillis. *Neuropsychological Rehabilitation, 3,* 235–244.

Baddeley, A. D., & Hitch, G. (1974). Working memory. In G. H. Bower (Ed.), *The psychology of learning and motivation* (Vol. 8, pp. 47–89). New York: Academic Press.

Baddeley, A. D., & Wilson, B. A. (1994). When implicit learning fails: Amnesia and the problem of error elimination. *Neuropsychologia, 32,* 53–68.

Barnes, M. (2016, May). *The cost of providing neurorehabilitation.* Paper presented at the World Congress of Neurorehabilitation, Philadelphia, PA.

Bateman, A. (2005). Life goals of people attending neuropsychological outpatient assessment after acquired brain injury. *Brain Impairment, 6,* 151–152.

Bateman, A., Teasdale, T. W., & Willmes, K. (2009). Assessing construct validity of the self-rating version of the European Brain Injury Questionnaire (EBIQ) using Rasch analysis. *Neuropsychological Rehabilitation, 19*(6), 941–954.

Bates, D. (2005). The vegetative state and the Royal College of Physicians guidance. *Neuropsychological Rehabilitation, 15*(3–4), 175–183.

Beck, A. T. (1976). *Cognitive therapy and the emotional disorders.* New York: International Universities Press.

Beck, A. T. (1996). Beyond belief: A theory of modes, personality, and psychopathology. In P. M. Salkovskis (Ed.), *Frontiers of cognitive therapy* (pp. 1–25). New York: Guilford Press.

Ben-Yishay, Y. (Ed.). (1978). *Working approaches to remediation of cognitive deficits in brain damaged persons* (Rehabilitation Monograph). New York: New York University Medical Center.

Ben-Yishay, Y. (1996). Reflections on the evolution of the therapeutic milieu concept. *Neuropsychological Rehabilitation, 6,* 327–343.

Ben-Yishay, Y., & Diller, L. (2010). *Handbook of holistic neuropsychological rehabilitation: Outpatient rehabilitation of traumatic brain injury.* New York: Oxford University Press.

Bennett, M., & Heard, R. (2010). Hyperbaric oxygen therapy for multiple sclerosis. *CNS Neuroscience and Therapeutics, 16,* 115–124.

Bennett, M., Trytko, B., & Jonker, B. (2012, December 12). Hyperbaric oxygen therapy for the adjunctive treatment of traumatic brain injury. Cochrane Database of Systematic Reviews, 2012, Article No. CD004609.

Bennett-Levy, J., Westbrook, D., Fennell, M., Cooper, M., Rouf, K., & Hackmann, A. (2004). Behavioural experiments: Historical and conceptual underpinnings. In J. Bennett-Levy, G. Butler, M. Fennell, A. Hackmann, M. Mueller, & D. Westbrook (Eds.), *Oxford guide to behavioural experiments in cognitive therapy* (pp. 1–20). Oxford, UK: Oxford University Press.

Berry, E., Kapur, N., Williams, L., Hodges, S., Watson, P., Smyth, G., . . . Wood, K. (2007). The use of a wearable camera, SenseCam, as a pictorial diary to improve autobiographical memory in a patient with limbic encephalitis: A preliminary report. *Neuropsychological Rehabilitation, 17,* 582–601.

Betteridge, S., Cotterill, E., & Murphy, P. (2017). Rehabilitation of challenging behaviour in community settings: The empowerment behavioural management approach (EBMA). In B. A. Wilson, J. Winegardner, C. van Heugten, & T. Ownsworth (Eds.), *Neuropsychological rehabilitation: The international handbook* (pp. 298–310). Abingdon, UK: Routledge.

Bigler, E. D. (2007). Traumatic brain injury and cognitive reserve. In Y. Stern (Ed.), *Cognitive reserve: Theory and applications.* New York: Taylor & Francis.

Bigler, E. D. (2012). Symptom validity testing, effort, and neuropsychological assessment. *Journal of the International Neuropsychological Society, 18,* 632–640.

Boake, C. (1996). Editorial: Historical aspects of neuropsychological rehabilitation. *Neuropsychological Rehabilitation, 6,* 241–243.

Boake, C. (2003). Stages in the history of neuropsychological rehabilitation. In B. A. Wilson (Ed.), *Neuropsychological rehabilitation: Theory and practice* (pp. 11–21). Lisse, the Netherlands: Swets & Zeitlinger.

Boussi-Gross, R., Golan, H., Fishlev, G., Bechor, Y., Volkov, O., Bergan, J., . . . Efrati, S. (2013). Hyperbaric oxygen therapy can improve post-concussion syndrome years after mild traumatic brain injury: Randomized prospective trial. *PLOS ONE, 8*(11), e79995. Retrieved from *http://journals.plos.org/plosone/article?id=10.1371/journal.pone.0174259.*

Bowen, A., Neumann, V., Conner, M., Tennant, A., & Chamberlain, M. A. (1998). Mood disorders following traumatic brain injury: Identifying the extent of the problem and the people at risk. *Brain Injury, 12,* 177–190.

Bower, G. H. (1972). Mental imagery and associative learning. In L. W. Gregg (Ed.), *Cognition in learning and memory* (pp. 51–88). New York: Wiley.

Boyle, M. E., & Greer, R. D. (1983). Operant procedures and the comatose patient. *Journal of Applied Behavior Analysis, 16,* 3–12.

Brewer-Mixon, K. K., & Callum, C. M. (2013). Historical principles and foundations of neuropsychological rehabilitation. In C. Noggle, R. Dean, & M. Barisa, *Neuropsychological rehabilitation* (pp. 1–11). New York: Springer.

British Medical Association (2017). Decisions to withdraw clinically assisted nutrition and hydration (CANH) from patients in permanent vegetative states (PVS) or minimally conscious states (MCS) following sudden-onset profound brain injury: Interim guidance for health professionals in England and Wales. Retrieved from *www.gmc-uk.org/end-of-life-care.*

British Psychological Society. (2011). *Good practice guidelines on the use of psychological formulation.* Leicester, UK: Author.

Broadbent, D. E., Cooper, P. F., Fitzgerald, P., & Parks, J. R. (1982). The Cognitive Failures Questionnaire (CFQ) and its correlates. *British Journal of Clinical Psychology, 21,* 1–16.

Browne, G., Berry, E., Kapur, N., Hodges, S., Smyth, G., Watson, P., & Wood, K. (2011). SenseCam improves memory for recent events and quality of life in a patient with memory retrieval difficulties. *Memory, 19,* 713–722.

Bruno, M. A., Bernheim, J. L., Ledoux, D., Pella, F., Demertzi, A., & Laureys, S. (2011). From unresponsive wakefulness to minimally conscious PLUS and functional locked-in syndrome: Recent advances in our understanding of disorders of consciousness. *Journal of Neurology, 258*(7), 1373–1384.

Bruns, J., & Hauser, W. A. (2003). The epidemiology of traumatic brain injury: A review. *Epilepsia, 44*(Suppl. 10), 2–10.

Buckley, N. A., Juurlink, D. N., Isbister, G., Bennett, M. H., & Lavonas, E. J. (2011, April 13). Hyperbaric oxygen for carbon monoxide poisoning. *Cochrane Database of Systematic Reviews, 2011*(4), Article No. CD002041.

Burgess, P. W., Alderman, N., Evans, J., Emslie, H., & Wilson, B. A. (1998). The ecological validity of tests of executive function. *Journal of the International Neuropsychological Society, 4,* 547–558.

Burton, C. R., Horne, M., Woodward-Nutt, K., Bowen, A., & Tyrrell, P. (2015). What is rehabilitation potential?: Development of a theoretical model through the accounts of healthcare professionals working in stroke rehabilitation services. *Disability Rehabilitation, 37*(21), 1955–1960.

Bütefisch, C. M. (2004). Plasticity in the human cerebral cortex: Lessons from the normal brain and from stroke. *Neuroscientist, 10,* 163–173.

Butler, G. (1998). Clinical formulation. In A. Bellack & M. Hersen (Eds.), *Comprehensive clinical psychology* (pp. 1–24). Oxford, UK: Pergamon Press.

Cahalan, S. (2012). *Brain on fire: My month of madness.* London: Allen Lane.

Caine, D., & Watson, J. D. G. (2000). Neuropsychological and neuropathological sequelae of cerebral anoxia: A critical review. *Journal of the International Neuropsychological Society, 6,* 86–99.

Camp, C. J., Bird, M., & Cherry, K. (2000). Retrieval strategies as a rehabilitation aid for cognitive loss in pathological aging. In R. D. Hill, L. Bäckman, & A. Stigsdotter-Neely (Eds.), *Cognitive rehabilitation in old age.* New York: Oxford University Press.

Caramazza, A. (1989). Cognitive neuropsychology and rehabilitation: An unfulfilled promise? In X. Seron & G. Deloche (Eds.), *Cognitive approaches in neuropsychological rehabilitation* (pp. 383–398). Hillsdale, NJ: Erlbaum.

Caramazza, A., & Hillis, A. E. (1993). For a theory of remediation of cognitive deficits. *Neuropsychological Rehabilitation, 3,* 217–234.

Cecatto, R. B., & Chadi, G. (2007). The importance of neuronal stimulation in central nervous system plasticity and neurorehabilitation strategies. *Functional Neurology, 22,* 137–143.

Christensen, A. L., & Teasdale, T. (1995). A clinical and neuropsychological led post-acute rehabilitation programme. In M. A. Chamberlain, V. C. Neuman, & A. Tennant (Eds.), *Traumatic brain injury rehabilitation: Initiatives in service delivery, treatment and measuring outcome* (pp. 88–98). New York: Chapman & Hall.

Christiansen, C. H., Huddleston, N., & Ottenbacher, K. J. (2001). Virtual reality in the kitchen. *American Journal of Physical Medicine and Rehabilitation, 80,* 597–604.

Cicerone, K. D., Langenbahn, D. M., Braden, C., Malec, J. F., Kalmar, K., Fraas, M., . . . Ashman, T. (2011). Evidence-based cognitive rehabilitation: Updated review of the literature from 2003 through 2008. *Archives of Physical Medicine and Rehabilitation, 92,* 519–530.

Cicerone, K. D., Mott, T., Azulay, J., Sharlow-Galella, M. A., Ellmo, W. J., Paradise, S., & Friel, J. C. (2008). A randomized controlled trial of holistic neuropsychologic rehabilitation after traumatic brain injury. *Archives of Physical Medicine and Rehabilitation, 89,* 2239–2249.

Clare, L. (2000). *Cognitive rehabilitation in early-stage Alzheimer's disease: Learning and the impact of awareness.* Unpublished doctoral thesis, Open University, Milton Keynes, UK.

Clare, L. (2008). *Neuropsychological rehabilitation and people with dementia.* Hove, UK: Psychology Press.

Clare, L., Bayr, A., Burns, A., Corbett, A., Jones, R., Knapp, M., . . . Whitaker, R. (2013). Goal-oriented cognitive rehabilitation in early stage dementia: Study protocol for a multi-centre single-blind randomised controlled trial (GREAT). *Trials, 14,* 152.

Clare, L., Wilson, B. A., Breen, E. K., & Hodges, J. R. (1999). Errorless learning of face–name associations in early Alzheimer's disease. *Neurocase, 5,* 37–46.

Clare, L., Wilson, B. A., Carter, G., Roth, I., & Hodges, J. R. (2002). Re-learning face–name associations in early Alzheimer's disease, *Neuropsychology, 16,* 538–547.

Coltheart, M. (1984). Editorial. *Cognitive Neuropsychology, 1,* 1–8.

Coltheart, M. (1991). Cognitive psychology applied to the treatment of acquired language disorders. In P. Martin (Ed.), *Handbook of behavior therapy and psychological science: An integrative approach* (pp. 216–226). New York: Pergamon Press.

Coltheart, M., Bates, A., & Castles, A. (1994). Cognitive neuropsychology and rehabilitation. In G. W. Humphreys & M. J. Riddoch (Eds.), *Cognitive neuropsychology and cognitive rehabilitation* (pp. 17–34). London: Erlbaum.

Cope, D. N., & Hall, K. (1982). Head injury rehabilitation: Benefit of early intervention. *Archives of Physical Medicine and Rehabilitation, 63*(9), 433–437.

Cowen, T. D., Meythaler, J. M., DeVivo, M. J., Ivie, C. S., Lebow, J., & Novack, T. A. (1995). Influence of early variables in traumatic brain injury on functional independence measure scores and rehabilitation length of stay and charges. *Archives of Physical Medicine and Rehabilitation, 76,* 797–803.

Crawford, C., Teo, L., Yang, E. M., Isbister, C., & Berry, K. (2017). Is hyperbaric oxygen therapy effective for traumatic brain injury?: A rapid evidence assessment of the literature and recommendations for the field. *Journal of Head Trauma Rehabilitation, 32,* E27–E37.

Cullen, B., Pownall, J., Cummings, J., Baylan, S., Broomfield, N., Haig, C., & Evans, J. J. (2016). Positive PsychoTherapy in ABI Rehab (PoPsTAR). *Neuropsychological Rehabilitation, 26,* 1–17.

Cullen, N. K., & Weisz, K. (2011). Cognitive correlates with functional outcomes after anoxic brain injury: A case controlled comparison with traumatic brain injury. *Brain Injury, 25*(1), 35–43.

Daisley, A., Tams, R., & Kischka, U. (2009). *Head injury: The facts.* Oxford, UK: Oxford University Press.

Davison, K. L., Crowcroft, N. S., Ramsay, M. E., Brown, D. W., & Andrews, N. J. (2003). Viral encephalitis in England, 1989–1998: What did we miss? *Emerging Infectectious Diseases, 9,* 234–240.

De Joode, E., Proot, I., Slegers, K., van Heugten, C., Verhey, F., & van Boxtel, M. (2012). The use of standard calendar software by individuals with acquired brain injury and cognitive complaints: A mixed methods study. *Disability and Rehabilitation: Assistive Technology, 7,* 389–398.

De Joode, E., van Heugten, C., Verhey, F., & van Boxtel, M. (2010). Efficacy and usability of assistive technology for patients with cognitive deficits: A systematic review. *Clinical Rehabilitation, 24,* 701–714.

Deluca, J. (2018, July). *New approaches to neurorehabilitation.* Paper presented at the International Neuropsychological Society Mid-Year Meeting: Bridging Science and Humanity, Prague, Czech Republic.

Dennis, M., & Kohn, B. (1975). Comprehension of syntax in infantile hemiplegics after cerebral hemidecortication: Left hemisphere superiority. *Brain and Language, 2,* 472–482.

Dewar, B. K., Kopelman, M., Kapur, N., & Wilson, B. A. (2015). Assistive technology for memory. In B. O'Neill & A. Gillespie (Eds.), *Assistive technology for cognition* (pp. 31–46). Hove, UK: Psychology Press.

Dewar, B. K., Pickard, J. D., & Wilson B. A. (2008). Long-term follow-up of 12 patients in the vegetative and minimally conscious states: An exploratory study. *Brain Impairment, 9,* 267–273.

Dhamapurkar, S., Wilson, B. A., Rose, A., & Florschutz, G. (2015). *Delayed recovery from the vegetative and minimally conscious states.* Poster presented at the 12th International Rehabilitation Congress, Daydream Island, Australia.

Diller, L. (1976). A model for cognitive retraining in rehabilitation. *The Clinical Psychologist, 29,* 13–15.

Diller, L. (1987). Neuropsychological rehabilitation. In M. Meier, A. Benton, & L. Diller (Eds.), *Neuropsychological rehabilitation* (pp. 3–18). New York: Guilford Press.

Dilley, M., Faiman, I., Goodliffe, L., Griffin, C., Smith, J., & Betteridge, S. (2017, March). *Neurorehabilitation service delivery changes: Effectiveness of hyperacute neurorehabilitation following traumatic brain injury.* Paper presented at National Health Service England's (NHSE) Pan London Providers Meeting, London, UK.

Ding, Z., Tong, W. C., Lu, X.-X., & Peng, H.-P. (2014). Hyperbaric oxygen therapy in acute ischemic stroke: A review. *Interventional Neurology, 2*(4), 201–211. Retrieved from *www.karger.com/Article/FullText/362677.*

Donaghy, M. (Ed.). (2011). Brain's diseases of the nervous system. In C. A. Noggle & R. S. Dean (Eds.), *The neuropsychology of cancer and oncology* (12th ed., pp. 1–12). New York: Springer.

Duckworth, A. L., Steen, T. A., & Seligman, M. E. P. (2005). Positive psychology in clinical practice. *Annual Review of Clinical Psychology, 1,* 629–651.

Duffau, H. (2006). Brain plasticity: From pathophysiological mechanisms to therapuetic applications. *Journal of Clinical Neuroscience, 13,* 885–897.

Duncan, J. (1986). Disorganization of behavior after frontal lobe damage. *Cognitive Neuropsychology, 3,* 271–290.

Easton, A. (2016). *Life after encephalitis: A narrative approach.* Hove, UK: Psychology Press.

Easton, A., & Hodgson, J. (2017). Encephalitis. In B. A. Wilson, J. Winegardner, C. van Heugten, & T. Ownsworth (Eds.), *Neuropsychological rehabilitation: The international handbook* (pp. 69–73). Abingdon, UK: Routledge.

Evans, J. J. (2009). The cognitive group: Part 1. Attention and goal management. In B. A. Wilson, J. J. Evans, F. Gracey, & A. Bateman (Eds.), *Neuropsychological rehabilitation: Theory, models, therapy and outcomes* (pp. 81–97). Cambridge, UK: Cambridge University Press.

Evans, J. J. (2011). Positive psychology and brain injury rehabilitation. *Brain Impairment, 12,* 117–127.

Evans, J. J., Emslie, H., & Wilson, B. A. (1998). External cueing systems in the rehabilitation of executive impairments of action. *Journal of the International Neuropsychological Society, 4,* 399–408.

Evans, J. J., & Krasny-Pacini, A. (2017). Goal setting in rehabilitation. In B. A. Wilson, J. Winegardner, C. van Heugten, & T. Ownsworth (Eds.), *Neuropsychological rehabilitation: The international handbook* (pp. 49–58). Abingdon, UK: Routledge.

Evans, J. J., & Williams, W. H. (2009). Caroline: Treating post-traumatic stress disorder after traumatic brain injury. In B. A. Wilson, J. J. Evans, F. Gracey, & A. Bateman (Eds.), *Neuropsychological rehabilitation: Theory, models, therapy and outcomes* (pp. 227–236). Cambridge, UK: Cambridge University Press.

Evans, J. J., & Wilson, B. A. (1992). A memory group for individuals with brain injury. *Clinical Rehabilitation, 6,* 75–81.

Evans, J. J., Wilson, B. A., Needham, P., & Brentnall, S. (2003). Who makes good use of memory-aids: Results of a survey of 100 people with acquired brain injury. *Journal of the International Neuropsychological Society, 9,* 925–935.

Fann, J. R., Hart, T., & Schomer, K. G. (2009) Treatment for depression after traumatic brain injury: A systematic review. *Journal of Neurotrauma, 26*(12), 2383–2402.

Farace, E., Alves, W. M. (2000). Do women fare worse?: A meta-analysis of gender differences in outcome after traumatic brain injury. *Journal of Neurosurgery, 93*(4), 539–545.

Fasotti, L. (2017). Mechanisms of recovery after acquired brain injury. In B. A. Wilson, J. Winegardner, C. van Heugten, & T. Ownsworth (Eds.), *Neuropsychological rehabilitation: The international handbook* (pp. 25–5). Abingdon, UK: Routledge.

Fish, J. (2017). Rehabilitation of attention disorders: Adults. In B. A. Wilson, J. Winegardner, C. van Heugten, & T. Ownsworth (Eds.), *Neuropsychological rehabilitation: The international handbook* (pp. 170–178). Abingdon, UK: Routledge.

Fish, J., Evans, J. J., Nimmo, M., Martin, E., Kersel, D., Bateman, A., . . . Manly, T. (2007). Rehabilitation of executive dysfunction following brain injury: "Content-free" cueing improves everyday prospective memory performance. *Neuropsychologia, 45,* 1318–1330.

Fish, J., Pamment, J., & Brentnall, S. (2017, July). *Training support workers to ensure continued rehabilitation success.* Datablitz presented at the Neuropsychological Rehabilitation Special Interest Group of the World Federation of Neurorehabilitation Meeting, Cape Town, South Africa.

Fish, J., Prince, L., & Winegardner, J. (2018, July). *"Finding the confidence to crack on with things": A qualitative study of client reflections on holistic neuropsychological rehabilitation several years post-programme.* Paper presented at the 15th annual conference of the Neuropsychological Rehabilitation Special

Interest Group for the World Federation of NeuroRehabilitation, Prague, Czech Republic.

Ford, C. L. (2017). Mood. In R. Winson, B. A. Wilson, & A. Bateman (Eds.), *The brain injury rehabilitation workbook* (pp. 204–234). New York: Guilford Press.

Forsyth, R. J., Wong, C. P., Kelly, T. P., Borrill, H., Stilgoe, D., Kendall, S., & Eyre, J. A. (2001). Cognitive and adaptive outcomes and age at insult effects after non-traumatic coma. *Archives of Disease in Childhood, 84,* 200–204.

Framingham, J. (2016). What is psychological assessment? *Psych Central.* Retrieved from *https://psychcentral.com/lib/what-is-psychological-assessment.*

Gainotti, G. (1993). Emotional and psychosocial problems after brain injury. *Neuropsychological Rehabilitation, 3,* 259–277.

Galton, F. (1907). *Inquiries into the human faculty and its development* (2nd ed.). New York: Dutton.

Gartland, D. (2004). Considerations in the selection and use of technology with people who have cognitive deficits following acquired brain injury. *Neuropsychological Rehabilitation, 14,* 61–75.

Gauggel, S., & Billino, J. (2002). The effects of goal setting on the arithmetic performance of brain damaged patients. *Archives of Clinical Neuropsychology, 17,* 283–294.

Gauggel, S., & Fischer, S. (2001). The effect of goal setting on motor performance and motor learning in brain-damaged patients. *Neuropsychological Rehabilitation, 11,* 33–44.

George, M., & Gilbert, S. (2018, May). Mental capacity act (2005) assessments: Why everyone needs to know about the frontal lobe paradox. *The Neuropsychologist, 5,* 59–66.

Giacino, J., & Whyte, J. (2005). The vegetative and minimally conscious states: Current knowledge and remaining questions. *Journal of Head Trauma Rehabilitation, 20,* 30–50.

Gianutsos, R. (1991). Cognitive rehabilitation: A neuropsychological specialty comes of age. *Brain Injury, 5,* 363–368.

Gilbert, P. (2009). *The compassionate mind.* London: Constable & Robinson.

Gilbert, P. (2010). *Compassion focused therapy: Distinctive features.* London: Routledge.

Gilbert, P., & Irons, C. (2005). Focused therapies and compassionate mind training shame and self-attacking. In P. Gilbert (Ed.), *Compassion: Conceptualisation, research and use in psychotherapy* (pp. 263–325). London: Routledge.

Glisky, E. L., & Schacter, D. L. (1986). Long-term retention of computer learning by patients with memory disorders. *Neuropsychologia, 26,* 173–178.

Glisky, E. L., Schacter, D. L., & Tulving, E. (1986). Computer learning by memory impaired patients: Acquisition and retention of complex knowledge. *Neuropsychologia, 24,* 313–328.

Goldstein, K. (1919). *Die behandlung, fürsorge und begutachtung der hirnverletzten (Zugleich ein beitrag zur verwendung psychologischer methoden in der klinik).* Leipzig, Germany: Vogel.

Goldstein, K. (1942). *After-effects of brain injuries in war: Their evaluation and treatment.* New York: Grune & Stratton.

Goodale, M. A., Milner, A. D., Jakobšon, L. S., & Carey D. P. (1990). Kinematic analysis of limb movements in neuropsychological research: Subtle deficits and recovery of function. *Canadian Journal of Psychology, 44,* 180–195.

GoPro. (2018). GoPro retrieved from *https://en.wikipedia.org/wiki/Gopro.*

Gracey, F., Evans, J. J., & Malley, D. (2009). Capturing process and outcome in complex rehabilitation interventions: A "Y-shaped" model. *Neuropsychological Rehabilitation, 19,* 867–890.

Granerod, J., Cousens, S., Davies, N. W. S., Crowcroft, N. S., & Thomas, S. L. (2013). New estimates of incidence of encephalitis in England. *Emerging Infectious Diseases, 19,* 1455–1462.

Granerod, J., & Crowcroft, N. (2007). The epidemiology of acute encephalitis. In B.-K. Dewar & W. H. Williams (Eds.), *Encephalitis: Assessment and rehabilitation across the lifespan* [Special issue]. *Neuropsychological Rehabilitation, 17,* 406–428.

Greenwood R. J., Strens, L. H. A., Watkin, J., Losseff, N., & Brown, M. M. (2004). A study of acute rehabilitation after head injury. *British Journal of Neurosurgery, 18,* 462–466.

Gross, Y., & Schutz, L. E. (1986). Intervention models in neuropsychology. In B. P. Uzzell & Y. Gross (Eds.), *Clinical neuropsychology of intervention* (pp. 179–205). Boston: Martinus Nijhoff.

Harris, R. (2009). *ACT made simple.* Oakland, CA: New Harbinger.

Hart, T. (2009). Treatment definition in complex rehabilitation interventions. *Neuropsychological Rehabilitation, 19,* 824–840.

Hart, T. (2017). Challenges in the evaluation of neuropsychological rehabilitation effects. In B. A. Wilson, J. Winegardner, C. van Heugten, & T. Ownsworth (Eds.), *Neuropsychological rehabilitation: The international handbook* (pp. 559–568). Abingdon, UK: Routledge.

Hart, T., Tsaousides, T., Zanca, J. M., Whyte, J., Packel, A., Ferraro, M., & Dijkers, M. P. (2014). Toward a theory-driven classification of rehabilitation treatments. *Archives of Physical Medicine and Rehabilitation, 95,* S33–S44.

Haslam, C., Holme, A., Haslam, S. A., Lyer, A., Jetten, J., & Williams, W. H. (2008). Group memberships for well-being after a stroke. *Neuropsychological Rehabilitation, 18,* 671–691.

Hayes, S. C. (2002). Acceptance, mindfulness, and science. *Clinical Psychology: Science and Practice, 9,* 101–106.

Hersch, N., & Treadgold, L. (1999). NeuroPage: The rehabilitation of memory dysfunction by prosthetic memory and cueing. *NeuroRehabilitation, 4,* 187–197.

Hessen, E., Nestvold, K., & Anderson, V. A. (2007). Neuropsychological function 23 years after mild traumatic brain injury: A comparison of outcome after paediatric and adult head injuries. *Brain Injury, 21,* 963–979.

Hodges, S., Berry, E., & Wood, K. (2011). SenseCam: A wearable camera that stimulates and rehabilitates autobiographical memory. *Memory, 19,* 685–696.

Hodgkinson, A. E., Veerabangsa, A., Drane, D., & McCluskey, A. (2000). Service utilization following traumatic brain injury. *Journal of Head Trauma Rehabilitation, 15*(6), 1208–1226.

Hossmann, K. A. (1999). The hypoxic brain: Insights from ischemia research. *Advances in Experimental Medicine and Biology, 474,* 155–169.

Houts, P. S., & Scott, R. A. (1975). *Goal planning with developmentally disabled persons: Procedures for developing and individual client plans.* Hershey: Department of Behavioral Science, Pennsylvania State University College of Medicine.

Hu, Q., Manaenko, A., Xu, T., Guo, Z., Tang, J., & Zhang, J. H. (2016). Hyperbaric oxygen therapy for traumatic brain injury: Bench-to-bedside. *Medical Gas Research, 6*(2), 102–110. Retrieved from *www.medgasres.com/article. asp?issn=2045-9912;year=2016;volume=6;issue=2;spage=102;epage=110;au last=Hu.*

Huang, L., & Obenaus, A. (2011). Hyperbaric oxygen therapy for traumatic brain injury. *Medical Gas Research, 1,* 21. Retrieved from *https://medicalgas-research.biomedcentral.com/articles/10.1186/2045-9912-1-21.*

Ince, L. P. (1976). *Behavior modification in rehabilitation medicine.* Baltimore: Williams & Wilkins.

Jamieson, M., Cullen, B., McGee-Lennon, M., Brewster, B., & Evans, J. J. (2014). The efficacy of cognitive prosthetic technology for people with memory impairments: A systematic review and meta-analysis. *Neuropsychological Rehabilitation, 24,* 419–444.

Jamieson, M., Cullen, B., McGee-Lennon, M., Brewster, S., & Evans, J. J. (2018, July). *Developing ApplTree: A smartphone reminding app for people with acquired brain injury.* Paper presented at the 15th annual conference of the Neuropsychological Rehabilitation Special Interest Group of the World Federation for NeuroRehabilitation, Prague, Czech Republic.

Jansari, A. S., Devlin, A., Agnew, R., & Akesson, K. (2014). Ecological assessment of executive functions: A new virtual reality paradigm. *Brain Impairment, 15,* 71–87.

Jennett, B. (1990). Scale and scope of the problems. In M. Rosenthal, E. R. Griffith, M. R. Bond, & J. D. Miller (Eds.), *Rehabilitation of the adult and child with traumatic brain injury* (pp. 3–7). Philadelphia: Davis.

Jennett, B., & Bond, M. (1975). Assessment of outcome after severe brain damage. *The Lancet, 1*(7905), 480–484.

Jetten, J., Haslam, C., & Haslam, S. A. (2012). *The social cure: Identity, health and well-being.* New York: Psychology Press.

Johansson, B. B. (2007). Regeneration and plasticity in the brain and spinal cord. *Journal of Cerebral Blood Flow and Metabolism, 27,* 1417–1430.

Johnson, D. A., Rose, F. D., Brooks, B. M., & Eyers, S. (2003). Age and recovery from brain injury: Legal opinions, clinical beliefs and experimental evidence. *Pediatric Rehabilitation, 6,* 103–109.

Judd, D., & Wilson, S. L. (2005). Psychotherapy with brain injury survivors: An investigation of the challenges encountered by clinicians and their modifications to therapeutic practice. *Brain Injury, 19,* 437–497.

Kabat-Zinn, J. (2013). *Full catastrophe living: How to cope with stress, pain and illness using mindfulness meditation.* London: Piatkus.

Kanfer, F. H. (1970). Self-regulation: Research issues and speculations. In C.

Neuringer & J. L. Michael (Eds.), *Behavior modification in clinical psychology* (pp. 178–220). New York: Appleton-Century-Crofts.

Kaplan-Solms, K., & Solms, M. (2018). *Clinical studies in neuro-psychoanalysis: Introduction to a depth neuropsychology* (2nd ed.). New York: Routledge.

Kapur, N., & Bradley, V. (2018). Neuropsychological interview. Retrieved from *http://londonmemoryclinic.com/wp-content/uploads/2018/06/interview-p.p.*

Kapur, N., Glisky, G. L., & Wilson, B. A. (2004). Technological memory aids for people with memory deficits. *Neuropsychological Rehabilitation, 14,* 41–60.

Keith, R. A., Granger, C. V., Hamilton, B. B., & Sherwin, F. S. (1987). The functional independence measure: A new tool for rehabilitation. *Advances in Clinical Rehabilitation, 1,* 6–18.

Keith, R. A., & Lipsey, M. (1993). The role of theory in rehabilitation assessment, treatment, and outcomes. In R. Glueckauf, L. Sechrest, G. Bond, & E. McDonel (Eds.), *Improving assessment in rehabilitation and health* (pp. 33–58). Newbury Park, CA: SAGE.

Kelly, G., Simpson, G. K., Brown, S., Kremer, P., & Gillett, L. (2017). The Overt Behaviour Scale—Self-Report (OBS-SR) for acquired brain injury: Exploratory analysis of reliability and validity. *Neuropsychological Rehabilitation, 27,* 1–19.

Kennard, M. A. (1940). Relation of age to motor impairment in man and subhuman primates. *Archives of Neurology and Psychiatry, 44,* 377–397.

Khan, F., Baguley, I. J., & Cameron, I. D. (2000). Rehabilitation after traumatic brain injury. *Medical Journal of Australia, 178,* 290–295.

Kime, S. K., Lamb, D. G., & Wilson, B. A. (1996). Use of a comprehensive program of external cuing to enhance procedural memory in a patient with dense amnesia. *Brain Injury, 10,* 17–25.

Kiresuk, T. J., & Sherman, R. E. (1968). Goal attainment scaling: A general method for evaluating comprehensive community mental health programs. *Community Mental Health Journal, 4*(6), 443–453.

Kiresuk, T. J., Smith, A., & Cardillo, J. E. (Eds.). (1994). *Goal attainment scaling: Applications, theory, and measurement.* Hillsdale, NJ: Erlbaum.

Kirsch, N. L., Levine, S. P., Fallon-Krueger, M., & Jaros, L. A. (1987). The microcomputer as an "orthotic" device for patients with cognitive deficits. *Journal of Head Trauma Rehabilitation, 2,* 77–86.

Kizony, R. (2011). Using virtual reality in cognitive rehabilitation. In N. Katz (Ed.), *Cognition, occupation and participation across the life span* (3rd ed., pp. 143–158). Bethesda, MD: AOTA Press.

Klein, O., Drummond, A., Mhizha-Murria, J., Mansford, L., & Das Nair, R. (2017). Effectiveness of cognitive rehabilitation for people with MS: A meta-synthesis of patient perspectives. *Neuropsychological Rehabilitation.* Retrieved from *www.ncbi.nlm.nih.gov/pubmed/28457198.*

Kleinrahm, R., Keller, F., Lutz, K., Kölch, M., & Fegert, J. M. (2013). Assessing change in the behaviour of children and adolescents in youth welfare institutions using goal attainment scaling. *Child and Adolescent Psychiatry and Mental Health, 7,* 33.

Klonoff, P. S., Stang, B., & Perumparaichallai, K. (2017). Family based support for people with brain injury. In B. A. Wilson, J. Winegardner, C. van Heugten, & T. Ownsworth (Eds.), *Neuropsychological rehabilitation: The international handbook* (pp. 364–377). Abingdon, UK: Routledge.

Knight, C., Alderman, N., Johnson, C., Green, S., Birkett-Swan, L., & Yorstan, G. (2008). The St Andrew's Sexual Behaviour Assessment (SASBA): Development of a standardised recording instrument for the measurement and assessment of challenging sexual behaviour in people with progressive and acquired neurological impairment. *Neuropsychological Rehabilitation, 18*, 129–159.

Kohn, B., & Dennis, M. (1978). Selective impairments of visuospatial abilities in infantile hemiplegics after right cerebral hemidecortication. *Neuropsychologia 12*, 505–512.

Kolb, B. B. (1995). *Brain plasticity and behaviour*. Hillsdale, NJ: Erlbaum.

Kurlychek, R. T. (1983). Use of a digital alarm chronograph as a memory aid in early dementia. *Clinical Gerontologist, 1*, 93–94.

Landauer, T. K., & Bjork, R. A. (1978). Optimum rehearsal patterns and name learning. In M. M. Gruneberg, P. E. Morris, & R. N. Sykes (Eds.), *Practical aspects of memory* (pp. 625–632). London: Academic Press.

Levin, H. S. (2003). Neuroplasticity following non-penetrating traumatic brain injury. *Brain Injury, 17*, 667–674.

Levine, B., Robertson, I. H., Clare, L., Carter, G., Hong, J., Wilson, M. A, . . . Stuss, D. T. (2000). Rehabilitation of executive functioning: An experimental–clinical validation of goal management training. *Journal of the International Neuropsychological Society, 6*, 299–312.

Lezak, M. D. (1988). Brain damage is a family affair. *Journal of Clinical and Experimental Neuropsychology, 10*, 111–123.

Lincoln, N. B. (1978). Behavioural modification in physiotherapy. *Physiotherapy, 64*, 265–267.

Lincoln, N. B., dasNair, R., Bradshaw, L., Constantinescu, C. S., Drummond, A. E. R., Erven, A., & Morgan, M. (2015). Cognitive rehabilitation for attention and memory in people with MS: Study protocol for a randomised controlled trial (CRAMMS). *Trials, 16*, 556. Retrieved from *www.ncbi.nlm. nih.gov/pmc/articles/PMC4672565*.

Lincoln, N. B., & Flannaghan, T. (2003) Cognitive behavioral psychotherapy for depression following stroke. *Stroke, 34*, 111–115.

Lincoln, N. B., Kneebone, I. I., Macniven, J. A. B., & Morris, R. C. (2012). *Psychological management of stroke*. Chichester, UK: Wiley.

Locke, E., & Latham, G. (2002). Building a practically useful theory of goal setting and task motivation. *American Psychologist, 57*, 705–717.

Logan, A., Oliver, J. J., & Berry, M. (2007). Growth factors in CNS repair and regeneration. *Progress in Growth Factor Research, 19*, 379–406.

Loveday, C., & Conway, M. A. (2011). SenseCam: The future of everyday memory research? *Memory, 19*, 1–124.

Luria, A. R. (1963). *Restoration of function after brain injury*. New York: Pergamon Press.

Luria, A. R. (1979). *The making of mind: A personal account of soviet psychology*. Cambridge, MA: Harvard University Press.

Ma, J., Zhang C.-G., & Li, Y. (2007). Bone marrow stromal cells transplantation for traumatic brain injury. *Journal of Clinical Rehabilitative Tissue Engineering Research, 11,* 2932–2935.

Maguire, E. A., Gadian, D. G., Johnsrude, I. S., Good, C. D., Ashburner, J., Frackowiak, R. S. G., & Frith, C. D (2000). Navigation-related structural change in the hippocampi of taxi drivers. *Proceeding of the National Academy of Sciences of the USA, 97,* 4398–4403.

Mahoney, F. I., & Barthel, D. (1965). Functional evaluation: The Barthel Index. *Maryland State Medical Journal, 14,* 56–61.

Malec, J. F. (2004). The Mayo–Portland Participation Index (M2PI): A brief and psychometrically-sound measure of brain injury outcome. *Archives of Physical Medicine and Rehabilitation, 85,* 1989–1996.

Malec, J. F. (2017). Assessment for neuropsychological rehabilitation planning. In B. A. Wilson, J. Winegardner, C. van Heugten, & T. Ownsworth (Eds.), *Neuropsychological rehabilitation: The international handbook* (pp. 36–48). Abingdon, UK: Routledge.

Manly, T., Heutink, J., Davison, B., Gaynord, B., Greenfield, E., & Parr, A. (2004). An electronic knot in the handkerchief: "Content free cueing" and the maintenance of attentive control. *Neuropsychological Rehabilitation, 14,* 89–116.

Manly, T., Robertson, I. H., Galloway, M., & Hawkins, K. (1999). The absent mind: Further investigations of sustained attention to response. *Neuropsychologia, 37,* 661–670.

Manning, K., McAllister, C., Ring, H., Finner, N., Kelly, C., Sylvester, K., . . ., Holland, A. (2016). Novel insights into maladaptive behaviours in Prader–Willi syndrome: Serendipitous findings from an open trial of vagus nerve stimulation. *Journal of Intellectual Disability Research, 60*(2), 149–155.

Mannion, A. F., Caporaso, F., Pulkovski, N., & Sprott, H. (2010). Goal attainment scaling as a measure of treatment success after physiotherapy for chronic low back pain. *Rheumatology, 49*(9), 1734–1738.

Markham, K. (2014). *Our time of day: My life with Corin Redgrave.* London: Oberon Books.

Marshall, J. F. (1985). Neural plasticity and recovery of function after brain injury. *International Review of Neurobiology, 26,* 201–247.

Max Planck Institute for Human Development and Stanford Center on Longevity. (2014). A consensus on the brain training industry from the scientific community. Retrieved from *http://longevity3.stanford.edu/blog/2014/10/15/the-consensus-on-the-brain-training-industry-from-the-scientific-community.*

Mayo Clinic. (2017). Brain aneurysm. Retrieved from *www.mayoclinic.org/diseases-conditions/brain-aneurysm/symptoms-causes/syc-20361483.*

McDonald, A., Haslam, C., Yates, P., Gurr, B., Leeder, G., & Sayers, A. (2011). Google Calendar: A new memory aid to compensate for prospective memory deficits following ABI. *Neuropsychological Rehabilitation, 21,* 784–807.

McGrath, J. C. (2008). Post-acute in-patient rehabilitation. In A. Tyerman & N. S. King (Eds.), *Psychological approaches to rehabilitation after traumatic brain injury* (pp. 39–64). Oxford, UK: Blackwell.

McMillan, T. M. (1996). Neuropsychological assessment after extremely severe head injury in a case of life or death. *Brain Injury, 11*(7), 483–490.

McMillan, T. M., & Greenwood, R. J. (1993). Models of rehabilitation programmes for the brain-injured adult–II: Model services and suggestions for change in the UK. *Clinical Rehabilitation, 7,* 346–355.

McMillan, T. M., & Herbert, C. M. (2004). Further recovery in a potential treatment withdrawal case 10 years after brain injury. *Brain Injury, 18*(9), 935–940.

McMillan, T. M., Teasdale, G. M., & Stewart, E. (2012). Disability in young people and adults after head injury: 12–14 year follow-up of a prospective cohort. *Journal of Neurology, Neurosurgery, and Psychiatry, 83,* 1086–1091.

McPherson, K. M., Kayes, N. M., & Kersten, P. (2017). MEANING as a smarter approach to goals in rehabilitation. In R. J. Siegert & W. M. M. Levack (Eds.), *Rehabilitation goal setting: Theory, practice and evidence* (pp. 105–119). Boca Raton, FL: CRC Press.

Menon, D. K., Schwab, K., Wright, D. W., & Maas, A. I. (2010). Position statement: Definition of traumatic brain injury. *Archives of Physical Medicine and Rehabilitation, 91,* 1637–1640.

Milieu Therapy. (2003) *Miller–Keane encyclopedia and dictionary of medicine, nursing, and allied health, seventh edition.* Retrieved from *https://medical-dictionary.thefreedictionary.com/milieu+therapy.*

Milieu Therapy. (2018). Retrieved from *https://en.wikipedia.org/wiki/Milieu_therapy.*

Miller, E. (1984). *Recovery and management of neuropsychological function.* Chichester, UK: Wiley.

Miller, J. D., Pentland, B., & Berrol, S. (1990). Early evaluation and management. In M. Rosenthal, E. R. Griffith, M. R. Bond, & J. D. Miller (Eds.), *Rehabilitation of the adult and child with traumatic brain injury* (2nd ed., pp. 21–51). Philadelphia: Davis.

Millis, S. R., Rosenthal, M., Novack, T. A., Sherer, M., Nick, T. G., Kreutzer, J. S., . . . Ricker, J. H. (2001). Long-term neuropsychological outcome after traumatic brain injury. *Journal of Head Trauma Rehabilitation, 16,* 343–355.

Mischel, W. (1968). *Personality and assessment.* New York: Wiley.

Mitchum, C. C., & Berndt, R. S. (1995). The cognitive neuropsychological approach to treatment of language disorders. *Neuropsychological Rehabilitation, 5,* 1–16.

Moffatt, N. (1989). Home-based cognitive rehabilitation with the elderly. In L. W. Poon, D. C. Rubin, & B. A. Wilson (Eds.), *Everyday cognition in adulthood and late life* (pp. 659–680). Cambridge, UK: Cambridge University Press.

Monti, M. M., Vanhaudenhuyse, A., Coleman, M. R., Boly, M., Pickard, J. D., Tshibanda, L., . . . Laureys, S. (2010). Willful modulation of brain activity in disorders of consciousness. *New England Journal of Medicine, 362*(7), 579–589.

Montour-Proulx, I., Braun, C. M. J., Daigneault, S., Rouleau, I., Kuehn, S., & Oégin, J. (2004). Predictors of intellectual function after a unilateral cortical lesion: Study of 635 patients from infancy to adulthood. *Journal of Child Neurology, 19,* 935–943.

Morris, R. (2018). Ethical issues and robotic or artificial intelligence care for people with neuropsychological conditions. *The Neuropsychologist, 5,* 40–42.

Mosch, S. C., Max, J. E., & Tranel, D. (2005). A matched lesion analysis of childhood versus adult-onset brain injury due to unilateral stroke: Another perspective on neural plasticity and recovery of social functioning. *Cognitive and Behavioral Neurology, 18,* 5–17.

Moyle, W. (2017). Social robotics in dementia care. In B. A. Wilson, J. Winegardner, C. van Heugten, & T. Ownsworth (Eds.), *Neuropsychological rehabilitation: The international handbook* (pp. 458–466). Abingdon, UK: Routledge.

Mozaffarian, D., Benjamin, E. J., Go, A. S., Arnett, D. K., Blaha, M. J., Cushman, M., . . . Turner, M. B. (2016). Heart disease and stroke statistics—2016 update: A report from the American Heart Association. *Circulation, 133*(4), e38–e360.

Nair, K. P. S., & Wade, D. T. (2003). Life goals of people with disabilities due to neurological disorders. *Clinical Rehabilitation, 17,* 521–527.

Nakase-Richardson, R., Sherer, M., Seel, R. T., Hart, T., Hanks, R., Arango-Lasprilla, J. C., . . . Hammond, F. (2011). Utility of post-traumatic amnesia in predicting 1-year productivity following traumatic brain injury: Comparison of the Russell and Mississippi PTA classification intervals. *Journal of Neurology, Neurosurgery and Psychiatry, 82,* 494–499.

NHS Trust v. Mr. Y and Mrs. Y (2018, July 30). [Supreme Court Ruling UKSC 46].

Norman, D. A. (1988). *The psychology of everyday things.* New York: Basic Books.

Nudo, R. J. (2013). Recovery after brain injury: Mechanisms and principles. *Frontiers in Human Neuroscience, 7,* 887.

Olsson, E., Wik, K., Ostling, A., Johansson, M., & Andersson, G. (2006). Everyday memory self-assessed by adult patients with acquired brain damage and their significant others. *Neuropsychological Rehabilitation, 16,* 257–271.

Olver, J. H., Ponsford, J. L., & Curran, C. A. (1996). Outcome following traumatic brain injury: A comparison between 2 and 5 years after injury. *Brain Injury, 10*(11), 841–848.

O'Neill, B., Jamieson, M., & Goodwin, R. (2017). Using technology to overcome impairments of mental functions. In B. A. Wilson, J. Winegardner, C. van Heugten, & T. Ownsworth (Eds.), *Neuropsychological rehabilitation: The international handbook* (pp. 434–446). Abingdon, UK: Routledge.

Owen, A. M., Coleman, M. R., Boly, M., Davis, M. H., Laureys, S., & Pickard, J. D. (2006). Detecting awareness in the vegetative state. *Science, 313*(5792), 1402.

Ownsworth, T. (2014). *Self-identity after brain injury.* Hove, UK: Psychology Press.

Ownsworth, T., & Gracey, F. (2017). Cognitive behavioural therapy for people with brain injury. In B. A. Wilson, J. Winegardner, C. van Heugten, & T. Ownsworth (Eds.), *Neuropsychological rehabilitation: The international handbook* (pp. 313–326). Abingdon, UK: Routledge.

Parr, A. M., Tator, C. H., & Keating, A. (2007). Bone marrow-derived mesen-chymal stromal cells for the repair of central nervous system injury. *Bone Marrow Transplantation, 40,* 609–619.

Patra, B. N., & Sarkar, S. (2013). Adjustment disorder: Current diagnostic sta-tus. *Indian Journal of Psychological Medicine, 35,* 4–9.

Peskine, A., Picq, C., & Pradat-Diehl, P. (2004). Cerebral anoxia and disability. *Brain Injury, 18,* 1243–1254.

Pinti, P., Aichelburg, C., Gilbert, S., Hamilton, A., Hirsch, J., Burgess, P., & Tachtsidis, I. (2018). A review on the use of wearable functional near-infrared spectroscopy in naturalistic environments. *Japanese Psychological Research, 60*(4), 347–373.

Playford, E. D., Siegert, R., Levack, W., & Freeman, J. (2009). Areas of con-sensus and controversy about goal setting in rehabilitation: A conference report. *Clinical Rehabilitation, 23*(4), 334–344.

Ponsford, J. (2013). Mechanism, recovery and sequelae of traumatic brain injury: A foundation for the REAL approach. In J. Ponsford, S. Sloan, & P. Snow (Eds.), *Traumatic brain injury: Rehabilitation for everyday adaptive living* (2nd ed.). Hove, UK: Psychology Press.

Ponsford, J., & Dymowski, A. (2017). Neuropsychological deficits and rehabili-tation following traumatic brain injury. In B. A. Wilson, J. Winegardner, C. van Heugten, & T. Ownsworth (Eds.), *Neuropsychological rehabilitation: The international handbook* (pp. 61–64). Abington, UK: Routledge.

Ponsford, J. L., Myles, P. S., Cooper, D. J., McDermott, F. T., Murray, L. J., Laid-law, J., . . . Bernard, S. A. (2008). Gender differences in outcome in patients with hypotension and severe traumatic brain injury. *Brain Injury, 39,* 67–76.

Poppelreuter, W. (1990). *Disturbances of lower and higher visual capacities caused by occipital damage: With special reference to the psychopathological, peda-gogical, industrial, and social implications* (J. Zihl & L. Weiskrantz, Trans.). Oxford, UK: Clarendon Press. (Original work published 1917).

Poser, U., Kohler, J. A., & Schönle, P. W. (1996). Historical review of neuropsy-chological rehabilitation in Germany. *Neuropsychological Rehabilitation, 6,* 257–278.

Premack, D. (1959). Towards empirical behavior laws: I. Positive reinforcement. *Psychological Review, 66,* 219–233.

Prigatano, G. P. (1986). Personality and psychosocial consequences of brain injury. In G. P. Prigatano, D. J. Fordyce, H. K. Zeiner, J. R. Roueche, M. Pepping, & B. C. Wood (Eds.), *Neuropsychological rehabilitation after brain injury* (pp. 29–50). Baltimore: Johns Hopkins University Press.

Prigatano, G. P. (1999). *Principles of neuropsychological rehabilitation.* New York: Oxford University Press.

Prigatano, G. P., Fordyce, D. J., Zeiner, H. K., Roueche, J. R., Pepping, M., & Wood, B. C. (Eds.). (1985). *Neuropsychological rehabilitation after brain injury* (p. 155). Baltimore: Johns Hopkins University Press.

Prince, L. (2017). Working with families after brain injury. In R. Winson, B. A. Wilson, & A. Bateman (Eds.), *The brain injury rehabilitation workbook* (pp. 263–276). New York: Guilford Press.

Rand, D., Basha-Abu Rukan, S., Weiss, P. L., & Katz, N. (2009). Validation of the Virtual MET as an assessment tool for executive functions. *Neuropsychological Rehabilitation, 19*, 583–602.

Rashid, T. (2015). Positive psychotherapy: A strength-based approach. *Journal of Positive Psychology, 10*, 25–40.

Raskin, S. A. (Ed.). (2011). *Neuroplasticity and rehabilitation*. New York: Guilford Press.

Ratcliff, J. J., Greenspan, A. I., Goldstein, F. C., Stringer, A. Y., Bushnik, T., Hammond, F. M., . . . Wright, D. W. (2007). Gender and traumatic brain injury: Do the sexes fare differently? *Brain Injury, 21*, 1023–1030.

Raymer, A., & Turkstra, L. (2017). Rehabilitation of language disorders in adults and children. In B. A. Wilson, J. Winegardner, C. van Heugten, & T. Ownsworth (Eds.), *Neuropsychological rehabilitation: The international handbook* (pp. 220–233). Abingdon, UK: Routledge.

Renison, B., Ponsford, J., Test, R., Richardson, B., & Brownfield, K. (2012). The ecological and construct validity of a newly developed measure of executive function: The Virtual Library Task. *Journal of the International Neuropsychological Society, 8*, 440–450.

Robertson, I. H. (1990). Does computerized cognitive rehabilitation work?: A review. *Aphasiology, 4*, 381–405.

Robertson, I. H. (1991). Book review. *Neuropsychological Rehabilitation, 1*, 87–90.

Robertson, I. H. (1996). *Goal management training: A clinical manual*. Cambridge, UK: PsyConsult.

Robertson, I. H. (2002). Cognitive neuroscience and brain rehabilitation: A promise kept. *Journal of Neurology, Neurosurgery and Psychiatry, 73*, 357.

Robertson, I. H., Manly, T., Andrade, J., Baddeley, B. T., & Yiend, J. (1997). "Oops!": Performance correlates of everyday attentional failures in traumatic brain injured and normal subjects. *Neuropsychologia, 35*, 747–758.

Robertson, I. H., & Murre, J. M. (1999). Rehabilitation of brain damage: Brain plasticity and principles of guided recovery. *Psychological Bulletin, 125*, 544–575.

Robertson, I. H., Ward, T., Ridgeway, V., & Nimmo-Smith, I. (1994). *The Test of Everyday Attention*. Bury St. Edmunds, UK: Thames Valley Test Company.

Robinson, F. B. (1970). *Effective study*. New York: Harper and Row.

Rockwood, K., Fay, S., Song, X., MacKnight, C., & Gorman, M. (2006). Attainment of treatment goals by people with Alzheimer's disease receiving galantamine: A randomized controlled trial. *Canadian Medical Association Journal, 174*(8), 1099–1105.

Roof, R. L., & Hall, E. D. (2000). Gender differences in acute CNS trauma and stroke: Neuroprotective effects of estrogen and progesterone. *Journal of Neurotrauma, 17*, 367–388.

Rose, F. D., Brooks, B. M., & Rizzo, A. A. (2005). Virtual reality in brain damage rehabilitation: Review. *Cyberpsychology and Behaviour, 8*, 243–251.

Royal College of Physicians. (2013). *Prolonged disorders of consciousness: National clinical guidelines*. London: Author.

Saez, M. M., Deakins, J., Winson, R., Watson, P., & Wilson, B. A. (2011). A ten-year follow up of a paging service for people with memory and planning problems within a healthcare system: How do recent users differ from the original users? *Neuropsychological Rehabilitation, 21,* 769–783.

Sahni, T., Jain, M., Prasad, R., Sogani, S. K., & Singh, V. P. (2012). Research reports—Use of hyperbaric oxygen in traumatic brain injury: Retrospective analysis of data of 20 patients treated at a tertiary care centre. *British Journal of Neurosurgery, 26,* 202–207. Retrieved from *www.ncbi.nlm.nih.gov/pubmed/22085249.*

Salkovskis, P. M. (Ed.). (1996). *Frontiers of cognitive therapy.* New York: Guilford Press.

Satapathy, M. C., Dash, D., Mishra, S. S., Tripathy, S. R., Nath, P. C., & Jena, S. P. (2016). Spectrum and outcome of traumatic brain injury in children <15 years: A tertiary level experience in India. *International Journal of Critical Illness and Injury Science,* 6(1), 16–20.

Schacter, D., & Crovitz, H. (1977). Memory function after closed head injury: A review of the quantitative research. *Cortex, 13,* 105–176.

Schönberger, M., Yeates, G. N., & Hobbs, P. (in press). Associations between therapeutic working alliance and social cognition in neurorehabilitation. *Neuropsychological Rehabilitation.*

Schutz, L. E. (2007). Models of exceptional adaptation in recovery after traumatic brain injury: A case series. *Journal of Head Trauma Rehabilitation, 22,* 48–55.

Seligman, M. E. P. (2011). *Flourish.* London: Nicholas Brearley.

Seligman, M. E. P., Steen, T. A., Park, N., & Peterson, C. (2005). Positive psychology progress: Empirical validation of interventions. *American Psychologist, 60,* 410–421.

Shah, U. (2017). Rehabilitation in India. In B. A. Wilson, J. Winegardner, C. van Heugten, & T. Ownsworth (Eds.), *Neuropsychological rehabilitation: The international handbook* (pp. 502–504). Abingdon, UK: Routledge.

Shiel, A. (1999). *Assessment and recovery of cognitive behaviours and cognitive impairment after severe traumatic brain injury.* Unpublished doctoral dissertation, University of Southampton, UK.

Shiel, A., Burn, J. P. S., Clark, D. H., Wilson, B. A., Burnett, M. E., & Mclellan, D. L. (2001). The effects of increased rehabilitation therapy after brain injury: Results of a prospective controlled trial. *Clinical Rehabilitation,* 15(5), 501–514.

Shiel, A., & Wilson, B. A. (1998). Assessment after extremely severe head injury in a case of life or death: Further support for McMillan. *Brain Injury, 12,* 809–816.

Shiel, A., Wilson, B. A., Horn, S., Watson, M., & McLellan, L. (1993). Can patients in coma following traumatic head injury learn simple tasks? *Neuropsychological Rehabilitation, 3,* 161–175.

Shiel, A., Wilson, B. A., McLellan, L., Horn, S., & Watson, M. (2000). *The Wessex Head Injury Matrix (WHIM).* Bury St Edmunds, UK: Thames Valley Test Company.

Siegert, R. J., & Levack, W. M. M. (Eds.). (2017). *Rehabilitation goal setting: Theory, practice and evidence.* Boca Raton, FL: CRC Press.

Simblett, S. K., Ring, H. A., & Bateman, A. (2017). The Dysexecutive

Questionnaire Revised (DEX-R): An extended measure of everyday dysexecutive problems after acquired brain injury. *Neuropsychological Rehabilitation, 27,* 1124–1141.

Sohlberg, M. M. (2006). External aids for management of memory impairment. In W. M. High, A. M. Sander, & M. A. Struchen (Eds.), *Rehabilitation for traumatic brain injury* (pp. 47–70). Oxford, UK: Oxford University Press.

Sohlberg, M. M., Johansen, A., Geyer, S., & Hoornbeek, S. (1994). *A manual for teaching patients to use compensatory memory systems.* Puyallup, WA: Association for Neuropsychological Research and Development.

Sohlberg, M. M., Kennedy, M., Avery, J., Coelho, C., Turkstra, L., Ylvisaker, M., . . . Yorkston, K. (2007). Evidence-based practice for the use of external aids as a memory compensation technique. *Journal of Medical Speech–Language Pathology, 15,* 15–51.

Sohlberg, M. M., & Mateer, C. A. (1989). *Introduction to cognitive rehabilitation: Theory and practice.* New York: Guilford Press.

Sohlberg, M. M., & Mateer, C. A. (2001). *Cognitive rehabilitation: An integrative neuropsychological approach.* New York: Guilford Press.

Stapley, S., Atkins, K., & Easton, A. (2009). *Acquired brain injury in adults (post encephalitis): A guide for primary and community care.* Malton, UK: Encephalitis Society.

Stein, D. G. (2007). Brain damage, sex hormones and recovery: A new role for progesterone and estrogen? *Trends in Neurosciences, 24,* 386–391.

Stein, D. G., & Hoffman, S. W. (2003). Concepts of CNS plasticity in the context of brain damage and repair. *Journal of Head Trauma Rehabilitation, 18,* 317–341.

Stern, Y. (2007). *Cognitive reserve: Theory and applications.* New York: Taylor & Francis.

Stone, M. J., & Hawkins, C. (2007). A medical overview of encephalitis [Special issue]. *Neuropsychological Rehabilitation, 17,* 429–449.

Stroke Association. (2017). Types of stroke. Retrieved from *www.stroke.org.uk/what-is-stroke/types-of-stroke.*

Sun, L., Perakyla, J., Holm, K., Haapasalo, J., Lehtimäki, K., Ogawa, K., . . . Hartikainen, K. (2017). Vagus nerve stimulation improves working memory performance. *Journal of Clinical and Experimental Neuropsychology, 39,* 954–964.

Sundberg, N. S., & Tyler, L. E. (1962). *Clinical psychology.* New York: Appleton-Century-Crofts.

Sunderland, A., Harris, J. E., & Baddeley, A. D. (1983). Do laboratory tests predict everyday memory?: A neuropsychological study. *Journal of Verbal Learning and Verbal Behavior, 22,* 341–357.

Swider, M. (2017, February 21). Google Glass review: Techradar. Retrieved from *www.techradar.com/reviews/gadgets/google-glass-1152283/review.*

Symonds, G. P. (1937). Mental disorder following head injury. *Proceedings of the Royal Society of Medicine, 30,* 1081–1094.

Tajfel, H., & Turner, J. (1979). An integrative theory of intergroup conflict. In W. G. Austin & S. Worchel (Eds.), *The social psychology of intergroup relations* (pp. 33–48). Monterey, CA: Brooks/Cole.

Tate, R. (2010). *A compendium of tests, scales and questionnaires: The practitioner's guide to measuring outcomes after acquired brain injury.* Hove, UK: Psychology Press.

Tate, R., & Perdices, M. (2017). Avoiding bias in evaluating rehabilitation. In B. A. Wilson, J. Winegardner, C. van Heugten, & T. Ownsworth (Eds.), *Neuropsychological rehabilitation: The international handbook* (pp. 547–558). Abingdon, UK: Routledge

Tate, R. L., Rosenkoetter, U., Vohra, S., Kratochwill, T., Sampson, M., Togher, L., ... Wilson, B. A. (2016). The Single-Case Reporting Guideline (BEhavioural Interventions [SCRIBE] 2016 statement). *Archives of Scientific Psychology, 4,* 1–9.

Tate, R., Simpson, G., Lane-Brown, A., Soo, C., de Wolf, A., & Whiting, D. (2012). Sydney Psychosocial Reintegration Scale (SPRS-2): Meeting the challenge of measuring participation in neurological conditions. *Australian Psychologist, 47,* 20–32.

Tate, R. L., Strettles, B., & Osoteo, T. (2003). Enhancing outcomes after traumatic brain injury: A social rehabilitation approach. In B. A. Wilson (Ed.), *Neuropsychological rehabilitation: Theory and practice* (pp. 137–169). Lisse, the Netherlands: Swets & Zeitlinger.

Tate, R., Taylor, C., & Aird, V. (2013). Applying empirical methods in clinical practice: Introducing the model for assessing treatment effect. *Journal of Head Trauma Rehabilitation, 28,* 77–88.

Taupin, P. (2006). Adult neurogenesis and neuroplasticity. *Restorative Neurology and Neuroscience, 24,* 9–15.

Teasdale, G., & Jennett, B. (1974). Assessment of coma and impaired consciousness: A practical scale. *The Lancet, 2*(7872), 81–84.

Teasdale, G., & Mendelow, D. (1984) Pathophysiology of head injuries. In N. Brooks (Ed.), *Closed head injury: Psychological, social and family consequences* (pp. 4–36). Oxford, UK: Oxford University Press.

Teasdale, T. W., Christensen, A.-L., Wilmes, K., Deloche, G., Braga, L., Stachowiak, F., ... Leclercq, M. (1997). Subjective experience in brain-injured patients and their close relatives: A European Brain Injury Questionnaire study. *Brain Injury, 11,* 543–563.

Thornton, M., & Travis, S. S. (2003). Analysis of the reliability of the modified Caregiver Strain Index. *Journals of Gerontology Series B: Psychological Sciences and Social Sciences, 58*(2), S127–S132.

Tobbel, J., & Burns, J. (1997). *Goal attainment scaling for people with learning disabilities.* Bicester, UK: Winslow.

Trexler, L. E., Parrott, D. R., & Malec, J. F. (2017). Replication of a prospective randomized controlled trial of resource facilitation to improve return to work and school after brain injury. *Archives of Physical Medicine and Rehabilitation, 97,* 204–210.

Trexler, L. E., Trexler, L. C., Malec, J. F., Klyce, D., & Parrott, D. R. (2010). Prospective randomized controlled trial of resource facilitation on community participation and vocational outcome following brain injury. *Journal of Head Trauma Rehabilitation, 25,* 440–446.

Turner-Stokes, L. (2012). *Goal attainment scaling (GAS): A practical guide.* London: Kings College.

Turner-Stokes, L., Bavikatte, G., Williams, H., Bill, A., & Sephton, K. (2016). Cost-efficiency of specialist hyper-acute in-patient rehabilitation services for medically unstable patients with complex rehabilitation needs: A prospective cohort analysis. *BMJ Open, 6*(9), e12112.

Turner-Stokes, L., Paul, S., & Williams, H. (2006). Efficiency of specialist rehabilitation in reducing dependency and costs of continuing care for adults with complex acquired brain injuries. *Journal of Neurology, Neurosurgery, and Psychiatry, 77*(5), 634–639.

Turner-Stokes, L., Pick, A., Nair, A., Disler, P., & Wade, D. (2015). Multidisciplinary rehabilitation for acquired brain injury in adults of working age. *Cochrane Database of Systematic Reviews,* Article No. CD004170.

Turner-Stokes, L., Williams, H., & Johnson, J. (2009). Goal attainment scaling: Does it provide added value as a person-centred measure for evaluation outcome in neurorehabilitation following acquired brain injury? *Journal of Rehabilitation Medicine, 41*(7), 528–535.

Turner-Stokes, L., Williams, H., Sephton, K., Rose, H., Harris, S., & Thu, A (2012). Engaging the hearts and minds of clinicians in outcome measurement: The UK rehabilitation outcomes collaborative approach. *Disability and Rehabilitation, 34*(22–23), 1871–1879.

Tyerman, A., & King, N. (2004). Interventions for psychological problems after brain injury. In L. H. Goldstein & J. McNeil (Eds.), *Clinical neuropsychology: A practical guide to assessment and management for clinicians* (pp. 385). Chichester, UK: Wiley.

van Heugten, C. M. (2017a). Stroke. In B. A. Wilson, J. Winegardner, C. van Heugten, & T. Ownsworth (Eds.), *Neuropsychological rehabilitation: The international handbook* (pp. 65–68). Abingdon, UK: Routledge.

van Heugten, C. M. (2017b). Novel forms of cognitive rehabilitation. In B. A. Wilson, J. Winegardner, C. van Heugten, & T. Ownsworth (Eds.), *Neuropsychological rehabilitation: The international handbook* (pp. 425–433). Abingdon, UK: Routledge.

van Heugten, C. M. (2017c). Outcome measures. In B. A. Wilson, J. Winegardner, C. van Heugten, & T. Ownsworth (Eds.), *Neuropsychological rehabilitation: The international handbook* (pp. 537–546). Abingdon, UK: Routledge.

van Heugten, C. M., Gregorio, G., & Wade, D. T. (2012). Evidence-based cognitive rehabilitation after acquired brain injury: Systematic review of content of treatment. *Neuropsychological Rehabilitation, 22,* 653–673.

van Heugten, C. M., Kessels, R. P. C., & Ponds, W. H. M. (2016). Brain training: Hype or hope? *Neuropsychological Rehabilitation, 26,* 639–644.

von Monakow, C. (1915). *Die Lokalisation im Grosshirn. Brain, 37,* 449–451.

Voss, H. U., Ülug, A. M., Dyke, J. P., Watts, R., Kobylarz, E. J., McCandliss, B. D., . . . Schiff, N. D. (2006). Possible axonal regrowth in late recovery from the minimally conscious state. *Journal of Clinical Investigation, 116,* 2005–2011.

Wade, D. T. (1999). Goal planning in stroke rehabilitation: What? *Topics in Stroke Rehabilitation, 6,* 8–15.

Wade, D. T. (2017). Foreword. In R. J. Siegert, & W. M. M. Levack (Eds.),

Rehabilitation goal setting: Theory, practice and evidence (pp. viii–ix). Boca Raton, FL: CRC Press.

Walsh, K. (1987). *Neuropsychology: A clinical approach*. Edinburgh, UK: Churchill Livingstone.

Weiss, P. L., Kizony, R., Feintuch, U., & Katz, N. (2006). Virtual reality in neuro-rehabilitation. In M. Selzer, S. Clarke, L. Cohen, G. Kwakkel, & R. Miller, *Textbook of neural repair and rehabilitation* (pp. 182–187). Cambridge, UK: Cambridge University Press.

Whitnall, L., McMillan, T. M., Murray, G. D., & Teasdale, G. M. (2006). Disability in young people and adults after head injury: 5–7 year follow up of a prospective cohort study. *Journal of Neurology, Neurosurgery and Psychiatry, 77*(5), 640–645.

Whyte, J. (1990). Mechanisms of recovery of function following CNS damage. In M. Rosenthal, E. R. Griffith, M. R. Bond, & J. D. Miller (Eds.), *Rehabilitation of the adult and child with TBI* (2nd ed.). Philadelphia: F. A. Davis.

Whyte, J. (1997). Distinctive methodological challenges. In M. J. Fuhrer (Ed.), *Assessing medical rehabilitation practices: The promise of outcomes research*. Baltimore: Brookes.

Williams, L. (2010, May 13). Sensecam human memory enhancement on BBC 2 TV Eyewitness [web log comment]. Retrieved from *www.youtube.com/watch?v=YAi2X6qf-4w*.

Williams, W. H., & Evans, J. J. (2003). *Neuropsychological rehabilitation*. Hove, UK: Psychology Press.

Williams, W. H., Evans, J. J., & Wilson, B. A. (1999). Outcome measures for survivors of acquired brain injury in day and outpatient neurorehabilitation programmes. *Neuropsychological Rehabilitation, 9*, 421–436.

Williams, W. H., Evans, J. J., & Wilson, B. A. (2003). Neurorehabilitation for two cases of post-traumatic stress disorder following traumatic brain injury. *Cognitive Neuropsychiatry, 8*(1), 1–18.

Wilson, B. A. (1991). Behaviour therapy in the treatment of neurologically impaired adults. In P. R. Martin (Ed.), *Handbook of behavior therapy and psychological science: An integrative approach* (pp. 227–252). New York: Pergamon Press.

Wilson, B. A. (1996a). Cognitive functioning of adult survivors of cerebral hypoxia. *Brain Injury, 10*, 863–874.

Wilson, B. A. (1996b). The ecological validity of neuropsychological assessment after severe brain injury. In R. J. Sbordone & C. J. Long (Eds.), *The ecological validity of neuropsychological testing* (pp. 413–428). Delray Beach, FL: GR Press/St. Lucie Press.

Wilson, B. A. (1997). Cognitive rehabilitation: How it is and how it might be. *Journal of the International Neuropsychological Society, 3*, 487–496.

Wilson, B. A. (1999). *Case studies in neuropsychological rehabilitation*. New York: Oxford University Press.

Wilson, B. A. (2002). Towards a comprehensive model of cognitive rehabilitation. *Neuropsychological Rehabilitation, 12*, 97–110.

Wilson, B. A. (2003a). The natural recovery and treatment of learning and memory disorders. In P. W. Halligan, U. Kischka, & J. C. Marshall (Eds.),

Handbook of clinical neuropsychology (pp. 167–180). Oxford, UK: Oxford University Press.

Wilson, B. A. (2003b). The future of neuropsychological rehabilitation. In B. A. Wilson (Ed.), *Neuropsychological rehabilitation: Theory and practice* (pp. 293–301). Lisse, the Netherlands: Swets & Zeitlinger.

Wilson, B. A. (2009). *Memory rehabilitation: Integrating theory and practice*. New York: Guilford Press.

Wilson, B. A. (2017). The development of neuropsychological rehabilitation: An historical examination of theoretical and practical Issues. In B. A. Wilson, J. Winegardner, C. van Heugten, & T. Ownsworth (Eds.), *Neuropsychological rehabilitation: The international handbook* (pp. 6–16). Abingdon, UK: Routledge.

Wilson, B. A., Allen, P., Rose, A., & Kubickova, V. (2018). *Locked-in syndrome after brain damage: Living within my head*. Abingdon, UK: Routledge.

Wilson, B. A., Baddeley, A. D., Evans, J. J., & Shiel, A. (1994). Errorless learning in the rehabilitation of memory impaired people. *Neuropsychological Rehabilitation, 4,* 307–326.

Wilson, B. A., Baddeley, A. D., Shiel, A., & Patton, G. (1992). How does posttraumatic amnesia differ from the amnesic syndrome and from chronic memory impairment? *Neuropsychological Rehabilitation, 2*(3), 231–243.

Wilson, B. A., & Bainbridge, K. (2014). Recovery takes time so don't give up. In B. A. Wilson, J. Winegardner, & F. Ashworth, *Life after brain injury: Survivors' stories* (pp. 50–62). Hove, UK: Psychology Press.

Wilson, B. A., Berry, E., Gracey, F., Harrison, C., Stow, I., MacNiven, J., . . . Young, A. W. (2005). Egocentric disorientation following bilateral parietal lobe damage. *Cortex, 41,* 547–554.

Wilson, B. A., Dhamapurkar, S. K., & Rose, A. (2016). *Surviving brain damage after assault: From vegetative state to meaningful life*. London: Routledge.

Wilson, B. A., Emslie, H., Quirk, K., & Evans, J. (1999). George: Learning to live independently with NeuroPage®. *Rehabilitation Psychology, 44,* 284–296.

Wilson, B. A., Emslie, H. C., Quirk, K., & Evans, J. J. (2001). Reducing everyday memory and planning problems by means of a paging system: A randomised control crossover study. *Journal of Neurology, Neurosurgery, and Psychiatry, 70,* 477–482.

Wilson, B. A., Evans, J., Brentnall, S., Bremner, S., Keohane, C., & Williams, H. (2000). The Oliver Zangwill Centre for Neuropsychological Rehabilitation: A partnership between health care and rehabilitation research. In A.-L. Christensen & B. P. Uzzell (Eds.), *International handbook of neuropsychological rehabilitation* (pp. 231–246). New York: Kluwer Academic/ Plenum.

Wilson, B. A., Evans, J. J., Emslie, H., & Malinek, V. (1997). Evaluation of NeuroPage: A new memory aid. *Journal of Neurology, Neurosurgery, and Psychiatry, 63,* 113–115.

Wilson, B. A., Evans, J. J., Gracey, F., & Bateman, A. (2009). *Neuropsychological rehabilitation: Theory, models, therapy and outcomes*. Cambridge, UK: Cambridge University Press.

Wilson, B. A., Evans, J. J., & Keohane, C. (2002). Cognitive rehabilitation: A goal-planning approach. *Journal of Head Trauma Rehabilitation, 17,* 542–555.

Wilson, B. A., Greenfield, E., Clare, L., Baddeley, A. D., Cockburn, J., Watson, P., . . . Nannery, R. (2008). *The Rivermead Behavioural Memory Test–3.* London: Pearson Assessment.

Wilson, B. A., & Jaramillo, J. D. (2014). Jose David's story: From medical student to medical anthropologist. In B. A. Wilson, J. Winegardner, & F. Ashworth (Eds.), *Life after brain injury: Survivors' stories* (pp. 63–74). Hove, UK: Psychology Press.

Wilson, B. A., Mole, J., & Manly, T. (2017). Rehabilitation of visual perceptual and visual spatial disorders in adults and children. In B. A. Wilson, J. Winegardner, C. van Heugten, & T. Ownsworth (Eds.), *Neuropsychological rehabilitation: The international handbook* (pp. 234–243). Abingdon, UK: Routledge.

Wilson, B. A., & Patterson, K. E. (1990). Rehabilitation for cognitive impairment: Does cognitive psychology apply? *Applied Cognitive Psychology, 4,* 247–260.

Wilson, B. A., Robertson, C., & Mole, J. (2015). *Identity unknown: How acute brain disease can affect knowledge of oneself and others.* Hove, UK: Psychology Press.

Wilson, B. A., Rous, R., & Sopena, S. (2008). The current practice of neuropsychological rehabilitation in the United Kingdom. *Applied Neuropsychology, 15,* 229–240.

Wilson, B. A., Scott, H., Evans, J., & Emslie, H. (2003). Preliminary report of a NeuroPage service within a health care system. *Neurorehabilitation, 18*(1), 3–8.

Wilson, B. A., & van Heugten, C. (2017). Neuropsychological deficits and treatment of survivors of cerebral hypoxia. In B. A. Wilson, J. Winegardner, C. van Heugten, & T. Ownsworth (Eds.), *Neuropsychological rehabilitation: The international handbook* (pp. 74–80). Abingdon, UK: Routledge.

Wilson, B. A., & Watson, P. C. (1996). A practical framework for understanding compensatory behaviour in people with organic memory impairment. *Memory, 4,* 465–486.

Wilson, B. A., Winegardner, J., & Ashworth, F. (2014). *Life after brain injury: Survivors' stories.* Hove, UK: Psychology Press.

Wilson, B. A., Winegardner, J., van Heugten, C., & Ownsworth, T. (Eds). (2017). *Neuropsychological rehabilitation: The international handbook.* Abingdon, UK: Routledge.

Winegardner, J. (2017) Executive functions. In R. Winson, B. A. Wilson, & A. Bateman (Eds.), *The brain injury rehabilitation workbook* (pp. 106–138). New York: Guilford Press.

Winegardner, J., & Fish, J. (2017, July). *A novel approach to interdisciplinary team assessment: Joining the dots.* Paper presented at the 14th international meeting of the Neuropsychological Rehabilitation Special Interest Group of the World Federation of NeuroRehabilitation, Cape Town, South Africa.

Winegardner, J., & Lodge, T. (2014). Tim's story: A seemingly mild injury just waiting to be understood. In B. A. Wilson, J. Winegardner, & F. Ashworth,

Life after brain injury: Survivors' stories (pp. 9–22). Hove, UK: Psychology Press.

Winson, R., Wilson, B. A., & Bateman, A. (Eds.). (2017). *The brain injury rehabilitation workbook*. New York: Guilford Press.

World Health Organization. (1980). *International classification of impairments, disabilities, and handicaps: A manual of classification relating to the consequences of disease.* Geneva, Switzerland: Author.

World Health Organization. (2001). *International classification of functioning, disability and health.* Geneva, Switzerland: Author.

Worthington, A., da Silva Ramos, S., & Oddy, M. (2017). The cost effectiveness of neuropsychological rehabilitation In B. A. Wilson, J. Winegardner, C. van Heugten, & T. Ownsworth (Eds.), *Neuropsychological rehabilitation: The international handbook* (pp. 469–479). Abingdon, UK: Routledge.

Ylvisaker, M., & Feeney, T. (2000). Reconstructing identity after brain injury. *Brain Impairment, 1,* 12–28.

Ylvisaker, M., Feeney, T. J., & Urbanczyk, B. (1993). Developing a positive communication culture for rehabilitation: Communication training for staff and family members. In C. J. Durgin, N. D. Schmidt, & L. J. Fryer (Eds.), *Staff development and clinical intervention in brain injury rehabilitation* (pp. 57–81). Gaithersburg, MD: Aspen.

Yule, W., & Carr, J. (1980). *Behaviour modification for the mentally handicapped.* London: Croom Helm.

Zangwill, O. L. (1947). Psychological aspects of rehabilitation in cases of brain injury. *British Journal of Psychology, 37,* 60–69.

Zarkowska, E. (1987). Discrimination and generalisation. In W. Yule & J. Carr (Eds.), *Behaviour modification for people with mental handicaps* (pp. 79–94). London: Croom Helm.

Zelviene, P., & Kazlauskas, E. (2018). Adjustment disorder: Current perspectives. *Neuropsychiatric Disease and Treatment, 14,* 375–381.

Zigmond, A. S., & Snaith, R. P. (1983). The Hospital Anxiety and Depression Scale. *Acta Psychiatrica Scandinavica, 67,* 361–370.

Index

The letter f after a page number indicates figure; the letter t indicates table.